body
Contouring

The

New

Art
_____
of

Liposculpture

Using Tumescent Local Anesthesia

William P. Coleman, III, M.D.
Clinical Professor of Dermatology, Tulane University Health Sciences Center
New Orleans, LA
  www.liposuctionneworleans.com

C. William Hanke, M.D., M.P.H., F.A.C.P.
Laser & Skin Surgery Center of Indiana, Indianapolis, IN
  www.cwmhanke.com

Rhoda S. Narins, M.D.
Clinical Professor of Dermatology,
New York University School of Medicine, New York, NY
  www.narins.com

William R. Cook, Jr., M.D.
Coronado, CA
  Retired

With Illustrations by Craig G. Gosling, CMI

Copyright © 2004, by Cooper Publishing Group LLC
Second edition

ALL RIGHTS RESERVED

No part of this publication may be reproduced, stored in a retrieval system, or transmitted, in any form or by any means, electronic, mechanical photocopying, recording, or otherwise, without the prior written permission of the publisher.

Library of Congress Cataloging in Publication Data:
    Coleman, William P.
    Body Contouring: The New Art of Liposculpture Using Tumescent Local Anesthesia

Cover Design: Gary Schmitt
Illustrations: Craig Gosling, and Gary Schmitt
                 Visual Media
                 Indiana University School of Medicine

Publisher: I. L. Cooper

Library of Congress Control Number: 2003114907

ISBN: 1-884125-99-9

Printed in the United States of America by Cooper Publishing Group LLC, P.O. Box 1129, Traverse City, MI 49685.

10 9 8 7 6 5 4 3 2 1

The Publisher and Author disclaim responsibility for any adverse effects or consequences from the misapplication or injudicious use of the information contained within this text.

For more information about this and other medical information titles, quantity purchase discounts, or to discuss new titles contact:
    Mr. I. L. Cooper, Publisher
    Cooper Publishing Group
    P.O. Box 1129, Traverse City, MI 49685
    (231) 933-9958
    E-mail: ICooper100@aol.com

Contents

Contributors

Craig G. Gosling, CMI
Professor Emeritus, Office of Visual Media, Indiana University School of Medicine, Indianapolis, IN

Michael F. Busk, M.D., M.P.H.
Medical and Research Director, National Institute for Fitness and Sport, Indianapolis, IN

Melanie A. Roberts, MS
Staff Exercise Physiologist and Director of the Fitness Center and the Center for Educational Services, National Institute for Fitness and Sport, Indianapolis, IN

Becky K. Zimmerman, R.D.
Formerly Staff Dietitian, National Institute for Fitness and Sport, Indianapolis, IN

Jane A. Rosemark, C.S.T.
Administrator, Laser & Skin Surgery Center of Indiana, Carmel, IN

Rene T. Guillotte, C.S.T.
Surgical Procedures Specialist, William P. Coleman III, M.D., Metairie, LA

Gary P. Schmitt
Graphic Design Image/Editing, Indiana University School of Medicine, Indianapolis, IN

Sarah P. Hanke, B.S.N., R.N., R.D.
Staff Nurse, Medical Intensive Care, Christ Hospital, Cincinnati, OH

Roberta Jacobs. B.A.
Surgical Procedures Specialist and Research Coordinator, Dermatologic Surgery and Laser Center, White Plains, NY

Preface

This book is dedicated to our patients. These individuals, like all of us, want to live healthy lives and look their best. In spite of a sound nutrition and exercise program (as outlined in Chapters 8 and 9), we all tend to develop localized body fat accumulations as we age. These fat accumulations are hereditary, and do not respond to diet and exercise. The accumulations are dependent upon the sex of the individual and are often seen in the majority of family members. The typical problem areas in women include the lower abdomen, upper outer thighs, upper inner thighs, hips, waist, buttocks, inner knees, arms and neck. The typical male problem areas include the upper abdomen, lower abdomen, waist (lovehandles), male breast enlargement (pseudogynecomastia), and neck.

Tumescent Liposculpture is a new method for permanently removing localized hereditary fat accumulations totally under local anesthesia. Several patient testimonials in Chapter 2 recount actual experiences with Tumescent Liposculpture. These individuals can now wear clothes that are one or more sizes smaller. They now feel better about themselves and their appearance. The self-image boost that occurs can have a very positive effect on the quality of one's life.

The illustrations that are seen throughout the book were drawn from actual patient photographs by Craig Gosling, Professor Emeritus, Office of Visual Media at Indiana University School of Medicine in Indianapolis, Indiana.

The chapter on nutrition was co-authored by Sarah Hanke and Becky Zimmerman. Melanie Roberts and Dr. Michael Busk co-authored the "On Your Way to Fitness" chapter. These recognized authorities are on the staff at the National Institute for Fitness and Sport (NIFS) in Indianapolis. We are also grateful to NIFS President, Mr. Jerry Taylor for his assistance.

The advice that is provided in the nutrition and exercise chapters is important for all of us whether we need Tumescent Liposculpture for localized hereditary adiposities or not. It is especially worthwhile to continue a healthy lifestyle following Tumescent Liposculpture in order to maximize and maintain improvement.

The chapter entitled "Most frequently asked questions about Tumescent Liposculpture" was prepared by Jane Rosemark and Rene Guillotte. Jane and Rene have extensive experience with Tumescent Liposculpture patients, and have answered these questions many times.

Lastly, a number of our patients and staff have reviewed drafts of this book at various stages of development. Their suggestions for improvement have been incorporated in the final manuscript. We cannot thank all of these talented people individually, but deeply appreciate their contributions.

> William P. Coleman III, M.D.
> C. William Hanke, M.D., M.P.H., F.A.C.P.
> William R. Cook, Jr., M.D.
> Rhoda S. Narins, M.D.

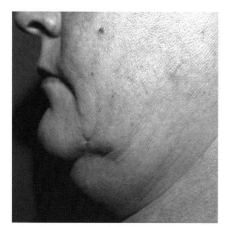 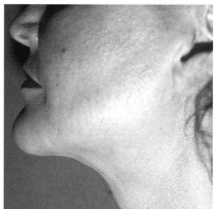

Used with permission, C. William Hanke, M.D.

Introduction

This book takes you on a fascinating journey through the world of

Tumescent Liposculpture, an advanced liposuction technique using only

tumescent local anesthesia designed to remove unwanted fat from the

body. The purpose of this book is to provide you with general

information. It is not meant to be a substitute for consultation with a

competent and caring cosmetic surgeon who specializes in Tumescent

Liposculpture. This book is also helpful for you to read and review after

consulting with your physician to gain a more complete education and

help you decide if Tumescent Liposculpture is right for you.

What Is Tumescent Liposculpture?

Tumescent Liposculpture is the advanced technique of permanently removing excess fat in areas which are resistant to diet and exercise using only Tumescent local anesthesia. It is called Tumescent (which means "to swell") because the surgeon "fills" and "swells" the fatty areas being removed with a special Tumescent solution before performing Liposculpture. This special Tumescent solution completely numbs the area with only local anesthesia. General anesthesia and intravenous ("IV") anesthesia are not needed and are not used, thus avoiding risks associated with them. The procedure is called Liposculpture because the surgeon is able to artistically sculpt the body into a new shape using Tumescent local anesthesia and smaller, more delicate instruments. This technique produces less bruising and less blood loss; offers a faster, safer, more comfortable recovery; and produces superior results compared to "old-style" liposuction performed under general or IV anesthesia. Tumescent Liposculpture has become a common procedure performed daily by cosmetic dermatologic surgeons throughout the United States.

History of "Old-Style" Liposuction and Tumescent Liposculpture

Prior to the 1970s, fat removal involved extracting blocks of fat through large skin incisions, resulting in long unsightly scars. In the mid-1970s, cosmetic surgeons in Italy and France began experimenting with a new method for removing excess fat. This technique became known as liposuction - literally suctioning out "lipo" or fat. The major goal of the surgeons was to utilize a cannula, a narrow tube with an opening on each end, to remove large amounts of fat through small incisions leaving less scarring. The cannula, which was attached to a suction device, was able to remove fat cells located beneath the skin. Areas as large as 100 square inches could be treated through one incision. By suctioning away the excess fat, a noticeable change in body contour was achieved. While the cannulas were an immediate improvement over large excisions of fat, the instruments were still large, general anesthesia was necessary, bleeding and bruising were profuse, and recovery was difficult and slow.

The most innovative approach to liposuction was developed by a dermatologist in the United States in 1987. This new form of liposuction, performed under local anesthesia, is known as Tumescent Liposculpture. Large volumes (1–5 liters) of a very dilute solution of local anesthesia and adrenalin were infused into the areas to be suctioned. This Tumescent solution not only provided the local anesthesia for the procedure but also allowed the patient to remain awake and comfortable throughout the procedure, avoiding the risks of general anesthesia. Other benefits of Tumescent Liposculpture over "old style" liposuction are the large amounts of the dilute adrenalin in the Tumescent solution which constrict the blood vessels, reducing bleeding and bruising to a minimum, and allowing the surgeon to spend more time shaping the areas for optimal results. Also, the Tumescent anesthesia provided a comfortable, rapid recovery, reducing the recovery time from weeks to only days. Now using this advanced approach, dermatologic surgeons could safely remove large amounts of fat, up to three to four liters (approximately six to eight pounds) per procedure, without general anesthesia and without significant blood loss. This was a dramatic improvement over "old-style" liposuction which required general anesthesia, and often led to blood transfusions, extensive bruising, and long recoveries. In fact, surgeons performing "old-style" liposuction routinely recommend transfusions of one unit of blood for every one-half liter of fat removed above one and one-half liters. In contrast, Tumescent Liposculpture does not require blood transfusions and bruising is minimal.

The goal of "old-style" liposuction was to just remove fat. With Tumescent Liposculpture, the dermatologic surgeon actually "sculpts" the body into a new, improved figure. Smaller, more delicate cannulas produce smoother contours and achieve superior tightening of the skin. Because there is almost no bleeding, the surgeon can take the time to sculpt the larger body areas into an improved figure.

Tumescent Liposculpture has been refined to a predictable safe approach now used all over the world. Because of the specialized Tumescent local anesthesia and the smaller cannulas, this new Liposculpture technique drastically decreases bleeding and bruising, allows greater comfort and safety for the patient, and provides superior results.

How Tumescent Liposculpture Works

Each person develops a certain number of fat cells by the end of puberty. These fat cells are "containers" which are filled with fat. The "containers" swell and shrink as a person gains and loses weight, but the number of "fat containers" remains the same. Certain body areas of localized excess fat have too many "containers" which may not shrink with diet and exercise. These areas are often hereditary. Family members often complain of localized fat deposits in the same body areas as their relatives. Parents and grandparents often have the same "problem areas." Although other areas of the body can be satisfactorily reduced, the "problem areas" resist diet and exercise. These "problem areas" usually include the abdomen, hips, buttocks, thighs, or neck, but can affect any area on both women and men.

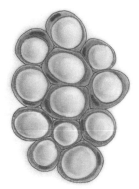

Figure 1-1. Fat cells are "containers" which are filled with fat. The cells increase and decrease in size as we gain and lose body weight.

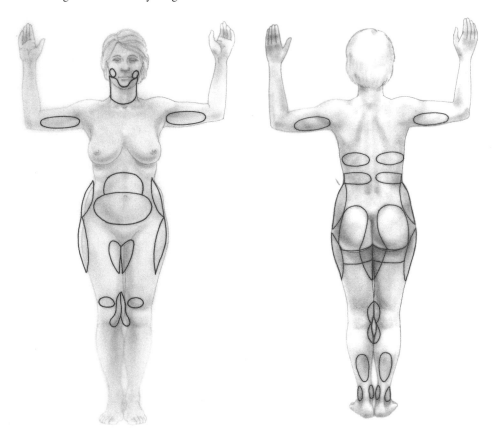

Figures 1-2 and 1-3. Typical hereditary localized problem areas in women include hips, outer thighs, abdomen, inner thighs, inner knees, buttocks, waist, calves/ankles, arms, and neck. Typical problem areas in men include abdomen, waist/love handles, breasts, and neck.

Most people realize that spot reducing of these "problem areas" cannot be achieved through diet or exercise. A person may lose weight, or tone muscle in certain areas, but the fat layer that covers these stubborn areas is resistant to all efforts. Tumescent Liposculpture provides the only reliable approach to spot reduction by permanently removing fat cells from the most difficult and resistant areas. Tumescent Liposculpture allows the physician to tunnel directly into the fatty layers of the body in a criss-cross pattern with fine cannulas, suctioning out the fat. A compression garment is worn after surgery to help the tunnels collapse and the skin to contour to its new shape.

Liposculpture is permanent because not only is fat removed, but the cells ("containers") that store the excess fat are also removed. Since new fat cells are not reproduced after they are removed, the suctioned areas do not re-expand. If a person gains weight after Liposculpture, the weight gain is distributed more evenly over the body rather than in the "problem areas" as before.

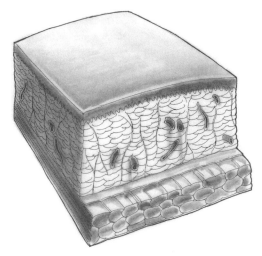

Figure 1-4. The subcutaneous fat layer under the skin is composed of many fat cells. Tiny blood vessels and nerves course through the fat.

6

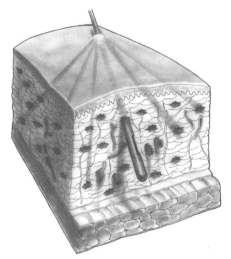

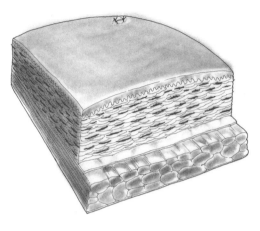

Figure 1-5. Following tumescent anesthesia, tunnels have been created in the fat with a small Liposculpture cannula.

Figure 1-6. The tunnels have collapsed following Tumescent Liposculpture. This ultimately results in a localized reduction of the thickness of the fat layer.

Who is a Candidate for Tumescent Liposculpture?

The ideal candidate for Liposculpture is a person who is in good health, exercises regularly, maintains good eating habits, and is within 25 pounds of his or her optimal weight.

A pinch test can determine whether a person can be helped by Liposculpture. A pinch test involves pinching the skin and fat between the thumb and index finger in order to determine the thickness of the tissue. Unless more than one inch can be pinched, Liposculpture may not be very useful. It is normal to have some fat beneath the skin in order to maintain a smooth appearance. Removing all of the fat beneath the skin would cause an irregular surface and an abnormal appearance.

People often mistake poor muscle tone for excess fat in some areas of the body. For example, sagging buttocks are often the result of poor development of the underlying muscles. Whether sagging buttocks is caused by excess fat or poor muscle tone can be determined by tensing the buttocks muscles tightly and pinching the overlying skin. If little skin can be pinched, then the answer is exercise, not Liposculpture. However, if more than one inch of skin and fat can be pinched with the buttocks tensed, Liposculpture may be indicated.

People should be realistic about the limitations of Liposculpture. Although Liposculpture can resculpt areas of excess fat, it cannot alter basic skeletal and muscular structure. If a person is large-boned, Liposculpture cannot change it. However, the excess fat over large hip bones can be removed to diminish the effect of large hips. During a consultation, the physician will explain the possible results that can be achieved by Liposculpture.

Liposculpture is not a treatment for generalized obesity. While fat can be removed from localized areas, obese people (those 20 percent over their recommended weight) should lose weight prior to or after Liposculpture. The suggested weight for adults is in Table 1-1 on page 11. Guidelines for nutrition and exercise programs are contained in Chapters eight and nine of this book.

Most people are good candidates for Liposculpture. However, certain medical conditions may limit one from having the procedure. Patients with severe heart, kidney, or liver disorders are not appropriate candidates for this procedure. Preoperative blood work is performed to confirm that the potential Liposculpture patient is in good health and has normal blood clotting ability.

Patients of almost any age can safely undergo Tumescent Liposculpture. Patients as young as 16 and as old as 80 have benefited from this procedure. Good results are much more dependent upon skin tone and activity level rather than biological age.

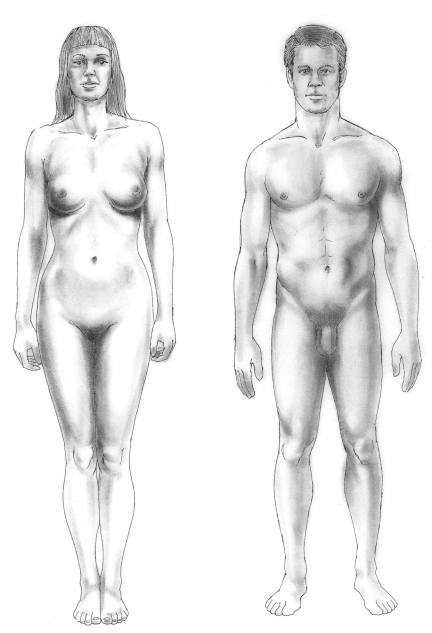

Figure 1-7. Idealized figure of a woman.   **Figure 1-8.** Idealized figure of a man

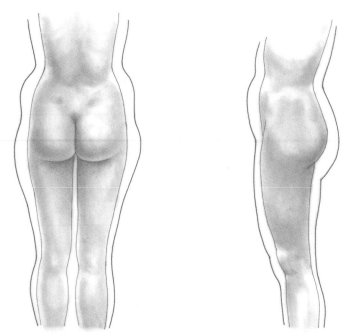

Figures 1-9 and 1-10. Tumescent Liposculpture can "turn back the clock" on a person's figure by reducing the thickness of the subcutaneous fat layer in selected body areas.

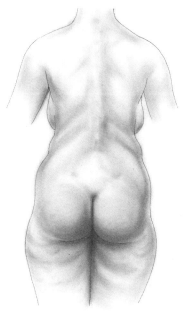

Figure 1-11. Excess fat deposits overlying the hips, outer thighs (saddlebags) and waist can develop as a woman ages.

Table 1-1. Weight chart

HEIGHT[1]	WEIGHT IN POUNDS[2]	
	to 34 years	35 years and over
5´0˝	97-128	108-138
5´1˝	101-132	111-143
5´2˝	104-137	115-148
5´3˝	107-141	119-152
5´4˝	111-146	122-157
5´5˝	114-150	126-162
5´6˝	118-155	130-167
5´7˝	121-160	134-172
5´8˝	125-164	138-178
5´9˝	129-169	142-183
5´10˝	132-174	146-188
5´11˝	136-179	151-194
6´0˝	140-184	155-199
6´1˝	144-189	159-205
6´2˝	148-195	164-210
6´3˝	152-200	168-216
6´4˝	156-205	173-222
6´5˝	160-211	177-228
6´6˝	164-216	182-234

[1]without shoes
[2]without shoes

The higher weights in the ranges generally apply to men, who tend to have more muscle and bone; the lower weights more often apply to women, who have less muscle and bone.

Source: Derived from National Research Council, 1989.

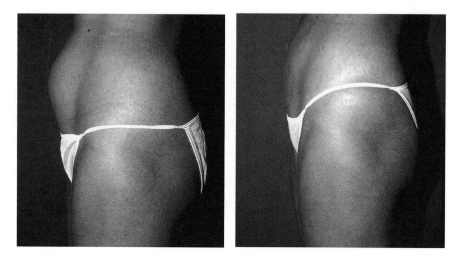

Used with permission, C. William Hanke, M.D.

Patients' Success Stories

The following are patients' true stories of their experiences with Tumescent Liposculpture.

Julia's Story

"Throughout adolescence, I was a competitive athlete in excellent physical condition, but I looked like a couch potato. I never felt like I looked as graceful on the balance beam as others did. A few years later it would be *Levi's*. Everyone wore them. I could get a pair on, but they looked hideous. And the beach, forget it. Styles come and go, but I only felt stylish in the late 1970s during the Annie Hall era of baggy men's pants. They hid the real me.

I can remember standing in front of our hallway mirror at age 11 and trying to imagine what it would be like to look 'normal.' My mother and I were both born with thunder-thighs, which are in fact 'normal' for the women in our family.

In 1987, I began reading articles about liposuction, making appointments and asking questions. I talked to doctors, nurses, surgeons, and friends. Finally, I scheduled a date for surgery. My dream was going to come true, but I started thinking about having a general anesthetic for elective surgery! Something was not right. Then my best friend, a nurse, sent me an article about the dangers of general anesthesia. The combination gave me cold feet and I backed out, but I did not forget my dream.

Then last fall I heard about Tumescent Liposculpture, using local anesthesia. At first I thought I was crazy! I'd just gone back to school for my master's degree and I was only working part-time. I vowed, however, that this time I was going to put myself first.

At the consultation I saw photos that showed the kind of change I was interested in for myself. Nothing would stop me now. I didn't tell friends and family who might try to change my mind, nor did I tell anyone who might not understand or judge this step negatively. I was definitely going through with it.

Tumescent Liposculpture was not only painless, I enjoyed it. I was making a dream come true. Now I stand in front of the aerobics class, not in back. I'm not a superficial person obsessed with my looks or with looking young. I rarely even wear make-up. But when I stood in a store, wearing a pair of jeans that I 'normally' would not have dared to even pick up, and turned around to look in the mirror and saw what I looked like from the back, I almost cried. I was so happy!"

Robert's Story

"I was 45 years old when I first looked into liposuction. However, I have been troubled by my 'love handles' since I was in my teens. Although I have gained and lost 10 pounds over and over, I have remained quite slender everywhere except for my love handles. I have always worked out regularly, but those bulges at my waist have never gone away. They are particularly difficult to disguise with clothes since they tend to hang over the top of my pants or bathing suits.

Although I had heard about Liposculpture for many years, I was not sure about this new procedure. Finally, I visited my dermatologic surgeon who I have known and trusted for many years. When I inquired about my love handles, I was surprised to hear how easily Liposculpture could help this problem. My doctor told me it could be done without general anesthesia and I would not have to go into the hospital. Although my enthusiasm began to build for getting rid of my love handles, I still did not believe that it could possibly be as easy as my doctor told me.

When I finally decided to have my Liposculpture, I anticipated my day of surgery with a mixture of fear and excitement. I was afraid that I would have pain or some other problem. But I was overwhelmed with excitement at the possibility of getting rid of my excess fat. On the day of my surgery, I was given a mild sedative to relax me and then a special local anesthesia fluid was gently placed into my waistline. My skin became quite firm and totally numb. As my fat was being suctioned, I only felt a mild pressure, like a massage, but no pain at all. I was able to talk to my doctor throughout the Liposculpture. In a short time my love handles were gone and I was able to stand up and already see immediate improvement!

That day, I rested in bed but felt no discomfort. The next morning I took a shower, went for a long walk and even went out for lunch. The areas operated on felt slightly bruised as if I had exercised too much. The next day I went back to work. Over the next couple of days, I gradually resumed my usual jogging.

I told my doctor that I had not totally believed him when he explained how easy Liposculpture could be. However, I had to admit to him afterwards that it was even easier than he had described. I could also hardy believe the immediate improvement in my waistline. My pants were looser almost immediately, and they kept getting looser over the next couple of months. It has now been more than a year since I had my Liposculpture. My only regret is that I didn't have it done years ago. My clothes fit better, I've gone down three inches, and I feel so much better in a bathing suit. I am even motivated to exercise more now that I look and feel so good. Tumescent Liposculpture is truly a miracle procedure."

Bridgette's Story

"My weight began to climb when I was in my thirties. By age 42 I had gained 20 pounds. Most of the weight went to my stomach and gave me a 'pot belly.' I looked three months pregnant in all of my clothes.

I tried to diet and exercise but I always became discouraged after a month or so because there would be some weight loss but the 'belly' remained.

The 'belly' began to undermine my self-image and I began to find myself more and more depressed over the way my stomach looked ... my 'belly' was all I saw when I looked into a mirror and my ability not to lose it became my greatest failure.

A friend told me about Tumescent Liposculpture and I immediately made an appointment with the doctor. After having the procedure explained to me in detail I set up an appointment for surgery.

In the weeks proceeding the surgery I told myself quite honestly that I did not care about the rest of the weight I had gained. All I wanted was this 'belly' removed. I had no desire to wear a bikini. All I wanted was to be able to zip my pants up.

The procedure was performed on an outpatient basis and the only medication I needed prior to the surgery was one Valium tablet. There was no pain during the procedure. In fact I have experienced greater pain when I have had my teeth cleaned. When I returned home I didn't even bother to have my pain prescription filled.

The outcome of the procedure was visible almost immediately. The 'belly' was gone and I was told (quite correctly) that my stomach would continue to 'shrink' for the next six months as the swelling from the suctioned tissue continued to vanish.

The most surprising result of Liposculpture was that once the 'belly' was gone I began to lose weight by simply maintaining the diet and moderate exercise program I had used previously. I have now lost 17 pounds.

Looking back, I realize that Tumescent Liposculpture is not the way to attain the perfect body, but rather a tool that can be used to attain a body that one can be comfortable and secure with. Once the results are visible from the Liposculpture procedure, then with attention to diet and exercise further fat reduction may be easier to achieve."

Greg's Story

"I am a fifty-eight year old man in excellent health and physical condition, successful in my profession, and confident personally and socially. There was perhaps only one thing that bugged me throughout my adult life and that was what is commonly referred to as 'love handles.' I had pockets of fat just above my hip bones on each side. Fortunately, the love handles were easily disguised under loose clothing. Unfortunately, there were still occasions in the locker room and at the beach when the love handles were exposed to the whole world.

All my life I have been actively engaged in sports and have worked out regularly. No matter how hard I tried, I could not get rid of the love handles. Because I was in great shape and not overweight, the love handles really were obvious, more so than they would have been on an overweight person. Long ago I had resigned myself to the fact that I would always have the love handles, but then one day I heard about Tumescent Liposculpture. At first I was skeptical that Tumescent Liposculpture could accomplish everything that the old-style Liposuction could without general anesthesia, the trauma, the blood loss, and the slow post-operative recovery. However, the more I investigated it, the more I was convinced I should give it a try.

The procedure was done on an outpatient basis. I actually walked out of the office to meet my wife waiting in the car. The procedure itself was a breeze, my pulse and blood pressure remained normal and I didn't need pain medicine that had been offered to me, since I had no pain or discomfort. I had a nice visit with my doctor and nurse during the procedure and even dozed off at one time.

I healed rapidly, the bruises and swelling were gone in a few weeks. Although the operative areas were slightly sore and there was some itching, there was no real pain and I never took so much as a Tylenol. Four weeks post-op no one in the locker room could tell I had surgery. Six weeks post-op I bared my new body to the beach crowd. While no one even suspected I had surgery, I did start receiving compliments. They were all to the effect that 'you sure look like you are in great shape.'

Needless to say, I am very pleased with the results of Tumescent Liposculpture and would have had it done years ago if it had been available. It is still hard to believe that I actually had it done but the mirror confirms it and the compliments from friends and family always bring a smile to my face. Tumescent Liposculpture was a quick fix for a life-long problem. My wife and I agree that life is too short and now is the time 'to go for it.' I did, and I might add that she did also and now looks better than she did 20 years ago. We could not be more pleased and now make an even greater effort to eat a nutritional, low fat diet, exercise regularly, and enjoy life to its fullest. Tumescent Liposculpture is a strong incentive to live a healthier life and maintain the best appearance possible as long as we live.

One year follow-up. It's been about a year since my Liposculpture and as my doctor predicted my body continues to reshape. All the tissue firmness has been absorbed and my waistline continues to slim down. The results are better than I had hoped. Tumescent Liposculpture is truly amazing. For those contemplating the procedure, I give the following advice:

1) Get involved in a moderate exercise program if you are not already doing so.
2) Good nutrition is essential including low fat foods and food supplements.
3) Don't eat as much.

I did all of the above and believe they played an important role in the great results of my Liposculpture. I have not gained any weight and feel better and look better than I have for years. I could not be more pleased."

Eight year follow-up. It has been 8 years since I had tumescent liposculpture. Although major back surgery has forced me to give up certain sports, I now swim almost every day to keep in shape and burn calories. My weight has dropped five pounds to 170 lbs. I look the same as I did, post surgery 8 years ago, except I have probably lost some muscle mass. My waist size has decreased from 34 inches to 32 inches and my "love handles" are still absent. My wife, who had a liposculpture procedure when I did, still looks as good as she did then as well. Neither of us have had any complications and I can't even find the tiny scars that used to be there. Tumescent liposculpture is a safe, simple and quick procedure that plays a role in our good self-image and happiness as we age. We agree that having tumescent liposculpture was a smart decision and we are glad we decided to do it. It was an investment that will last as long as we live.

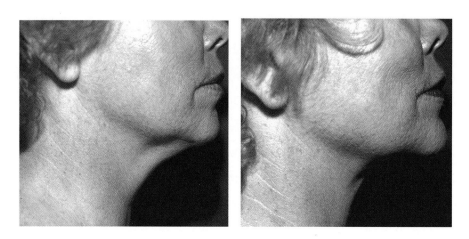

Used with permission, C. William Hanke, M.D.

Tumescent Liposculpture for Different Areas of the Body

Nearly every part of the body can benefit from Liposculpture. Patients may choose to have one or more areas sculpted at the same time. To achieve your optimal shape, your physician may suggest treating various combinations of body areas that will give you the best figure.

The Face, Neck, and Jowls

With age, there is a natural tendency to accumulate excess fat in the lower face and neck. This is particularly pronounced in some individuals due to heredity, and is commonly known as a "turkey neck." Fortunately, Liposculpture is successful in improving this problem. Excess fat in the lower face causes bulging of the overlying skin and eventual drooping of facial tissue causing jowls. However, in most individuals, conservative Liposculpture of the excess fat of the lower face, jowls, and neck can tighten the skin so that a face-lift can be avoided or delayed. Tumescent Liposculpture of the lower face, jowls, and neck often makes the face and neck appear 10 years younger. Even individuals with large fatty necks can achieve considerable benefits from Liposculpture. Dramatic improvement is often apparent within a few weeks after surgery. Patients can have Liposculpture on Friday and return to work on Monday looking younger and "thinner" without the tell-tale signs of surgery. If there is loose skin or muscle under the chin, it can be improved by a simple neck lift procedure.

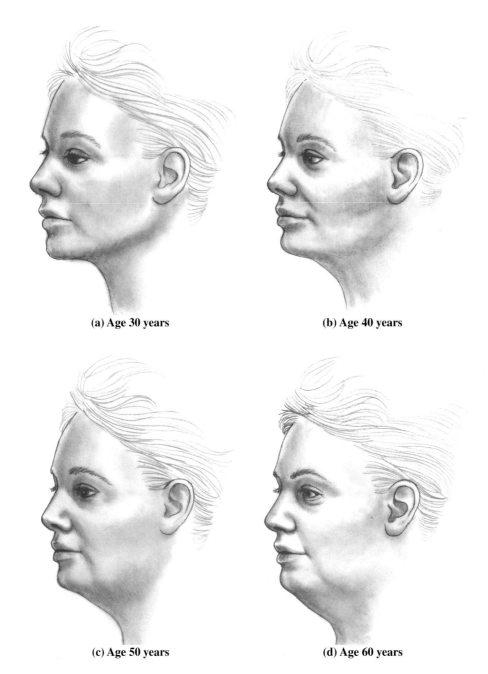

(a) Age 30 years   **(b) Age 40 years**

(c) Age 50 years   **(d) Age 60 years**

Figure 3-1. Heredity is the major determinant of fat deposition in the neck. Fat accumulations in the neck may worsen progressively with age. Some individuals have a hereditary predisposition to develop fat in the neck by the age of 20 or 30 years. Tumescent Liposculpture of the neck can lead to dramatic improvement in appearance and self-esteem.

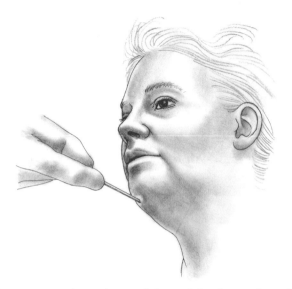

Figure 3-2. Tumescent Liposculpture of the neck is often performed through tiny incisions underneath the chin and below each ear.

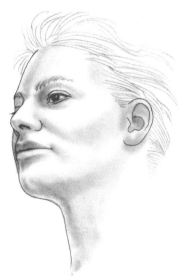

Figure 3-3 A firmer, younger-looking neck is present following Tumescent Liposculpture.

The Arms

Some people accumulate excess fat on the back of the arms. This often occurs after numerous gains and losses in weight and has a strong genetic tendency, "like mother, like daughter." In many cases this can be corrected by Liposculpture. Excess fat is removed from the back of the entire upper arm. This allows the skin to tighten, leaving the arms slimmer and more attractive.

The Abdomen

When most people think of fat, they think of the abdominal area. Many individuals have a tendency to accumulate most of their excess fat in the upper and lower abdomen. The abdomen is a common problem area for both men and women. Liposculpture can assist with this problem, even for people with enormous accumulations of fat in their abdomen. Liposculpture cannot correct poor muscle tone. In these cases, sometimes a "tummy tuck" or abdominoplasty is required to achieve full correction. However, many people who think they need a "tummy tuck" are actually excellent candidates for Liposculpture alone. Liposculpture is less invasive, does not require general anesthesia, does not leave the 10 or 20 inch scar of a "tummy tuck," requires less recovery time, and can often provide the desired benefits easily and safely.

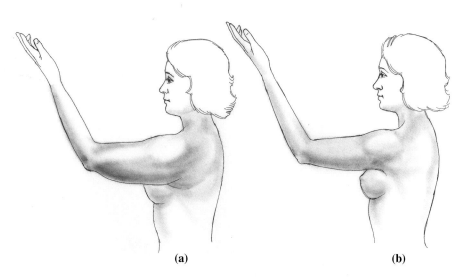

(a)   (b)

Figure 3-4. (a) Women may develop hereditary fat accumulations on the back of the arms. **(b)** The arm has a more normal contour following Tumescent Liposculpture.

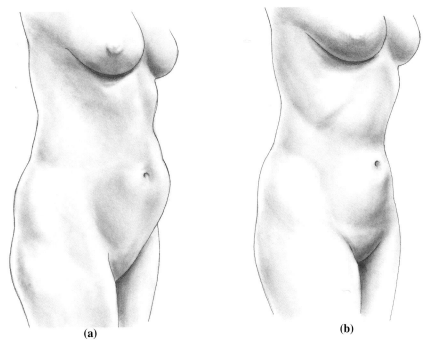

(a)   (b)

Figure 3-5. (a) Some women have a hereditary tendency to develop fat accumulations on the abdomen as they age. **(b)** A more pleasing abdominal contour has been achieved following Tumescent Liposculpture.

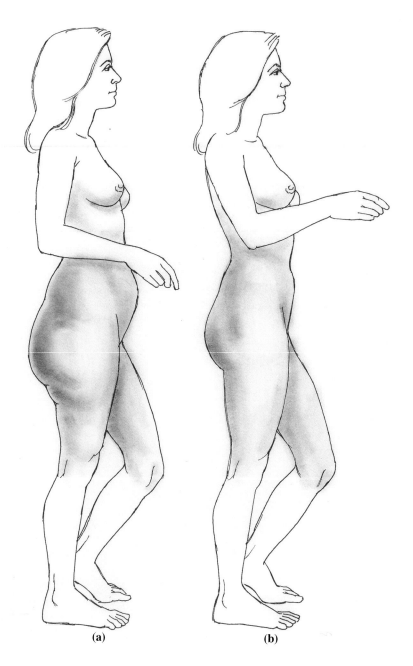

(a)   (b)

Figure 3-6. (a) Some patients develop localized, hereditary fat deposits in multiple areas including the abdomen, hips and buttocks. **(b)** The figure has been trimmed following Tumescent Liposculpture.

Breast, Chest, and Bulges Around Underarms

Men and boys may have excess fat in the chest area which resembles female breasts. Some men are embarrassed to wear tight shirts or to remove their shirts in public. This excess fat can be removed successfully with Tumescent Liposculpture.

Excess fat that bulges in front of and just behind the underarms also can be removed in both men and women. Liposculpture of these areas gives a firmer, more trim appearance to the chest and upper back.

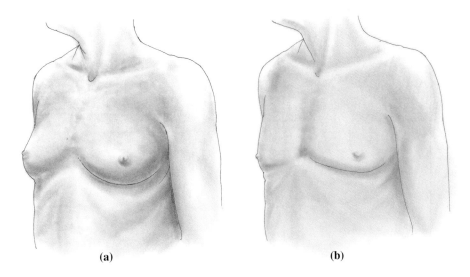

(a)   (b)

Figure 3-7. (a) Some men develop large deposits of subcutaneous fat in the breasts. **(b)** Removal of fat using Tumescent Liposculpture can create a more normal appearance. Women with large breasts can have them reduced in size by undergoing Tumescent Liposculpture. This method is preferred over traditional breast reduction because it leaves no scars. However, only modest changes in breast size can be achieved using Liposculpture.

Waist, Flanks, and Hips

Men commonly accumulate excess fat in the flanks or "love handle" areas even if they are not overweight and exercise regularly. Women often develop undesirable fat deposits on the hips just over the hip bone. Some women even "lose their waists" to excess fat. All of these problem areas are correctable by Tumescent Liposculpture. Liposculpture of these areas may result in a considerable reduction in waist measurement, commonly as much as two to six inches, and allows a much better fit for form-fitting clothes. Many patients are pleased to find they can wear clothing one or more sizes smaller and have a younger looking physique.

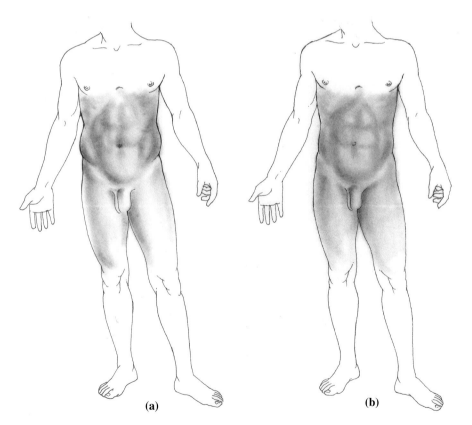

(a)   (b)

Figure 3-8. (a) Men often develop localized fat in the waist/love handle area. **(b)** A trimmer waist is achieved through Tumescent Liposculpture.

Back

Excess fat may accumulate in folds on the mid-back or just behind the underarms. In women, this can lead to bulging in and around the bra strap.

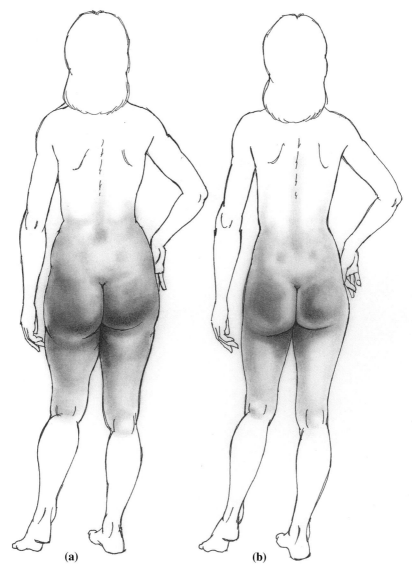

(a)   **(b)**

Figure 3-9. (a) Women can develop large deposits of fat on the hips on a hereditary basis.
(b) Tumescent Liposculpture can remove the localized fat accumulations.

People often find these excess bulges and folds unattractive since they can be seen through clothing. Liposculpture can successfully recontour these areas. Clothes usually fit more comfortably after Liposculpture.

Buttocks

Women may accumulate excess fat in the buttocks as they age. Many women who perceive that they have "saddle bags" actually have excess fat in the buttocks - the buttocks sag and bulge over the thigh areas. In these cases Liposculpture of the buttocks alone (without much work on the thighs) can provide an excellent result. Liposculpture of the buttocks is primarily performed on the outer-two-thirds so as not to flatten the central buttocks. Some people also accumulate a small area of excess fat in the upper part of the buttocks where it meets the lower back. Liposculpture is an excellent technique for reducing this area.

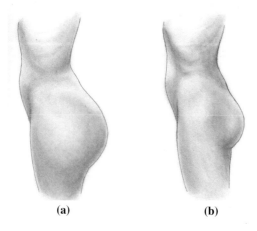

(a)   (b)

Figure 3-10. (a) Some individuals develop enlargement of the buttocks with age. **(b)** Tumescent Liposculpture can remove the localized fat accumulations.

Outer Thighs

Some people have a natural tendency for excess fat to accumulate on the outer thighs. This gives the illusion of riding breeches or so-called "saddle bags." The fullness first begins in the teen-age years and may progress to a major figure problem in adulthood. Although many hours can be spent exercising the outer thighs, this area is usually resistant to reduction by any method other than Liposculpture. Tumescent Liposculpture is the ideal approach for recontouring the outer thighs and has been used successfully in hundreds of thousands of people.

Liposculpture of the outer thighs is often combined with that of the buttocks to achieve the best figure improvement. Liposculpture can be performed around the entire thigh to reduce the diameter of the entire leg, usually in two sessions.

Some individuals are slender from the waist up and yet have large thighs and buttocks. Liposculpture can give them a more symmetrical figure.

Inner Thighs

Some individuals develop accumulations of excess fat in the inner thighs. The thighs may even rub together. This is not only unattractive but uncomfortable. Liposculpture can remove the excess fat, resulting in a slimming of the thighs and more attractive legs.

Back of Thighs

Another common area where excess fat accumulates is beneath the buttocks, over the back of the thighs with irregularities or dimpling of the skin. This cottage cheese appearance can be improved using the smaller cannulas during Tumescent Liposculpture, resulting in a smoother, better contour. Fat that collects beneath the buttocks (called the banana roll) can also be sculpted for a

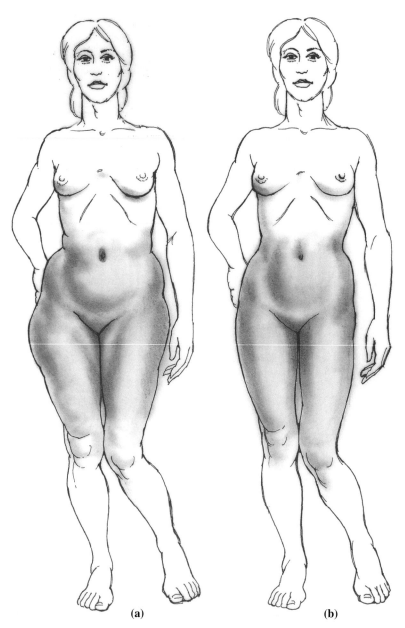

Figure 3-11. (a) Women may develop fat accumulations on the outer thighs, hips and inner thighs. **(b)** Tumescent Liposculpture can slim these areas.

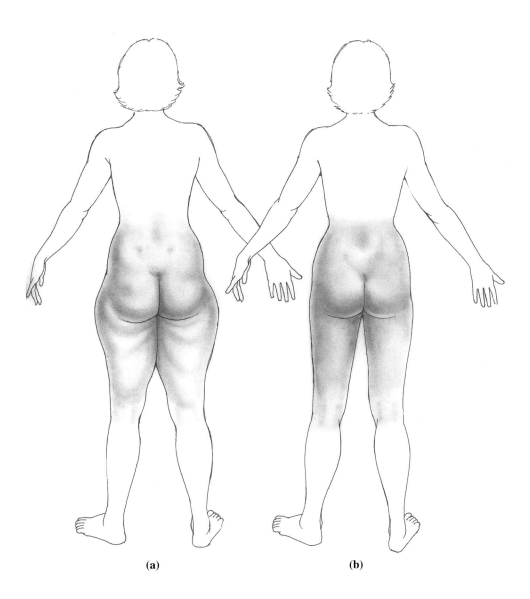

(a)   (b)

Figure 3-12. (a) Women may develop fat accumulations on the outer thighs, hips and inner thighs. **(b)** Tumescent Liposculpture can slim these areas.

firmer, flatter appearance. Tumescent Liposculpture of the back of the thighs may be combined with Liposculpture of the buttocks, outer thighs, or inner thighs.

Front and Inner Thighs

A common hereditary tendency is seen in people with excess fat on the front and inner area of the thighs. This area can become so heavy that it starts to hang over the knees and the thighs can even rub together. Tumescent Liposculpture can be used for these areas and results in more shapely thighs, revealing the underlying muscle definition. Liposculpture of the front and inner thighs is often combined with Liposculpture of the knees.

Knees

Fat may accumulate on the inside of the knees and/or just below the kneecap. Both of these areas can be corrected by Liposculpture. In some cases, the accumulation on the inside is severe enough to cause the knees to rub together, leading to discomfort. In other cases, only a small amount of fat resides here but is enough to distort the contour of the legs. Many people think they have ugly knees due to large underlying bone structures. These individuals are surprised to find that Tumescent Liposculpture can give them slimmer knees and a more athletic look to the leg.

Calves and Ankles

In addition to the knees, individuals may also accumulate excess fat around the lower calf and ankle area to give them a "peg leg" or "piano leg" appearance. Liposculpture can be used in the calf and around the ankles to reduce the excess fat. This defines the calf muscles resulting in much more attractive legs and ankles. Shoes and boots often fit much better following Tumescent Liposculpture.

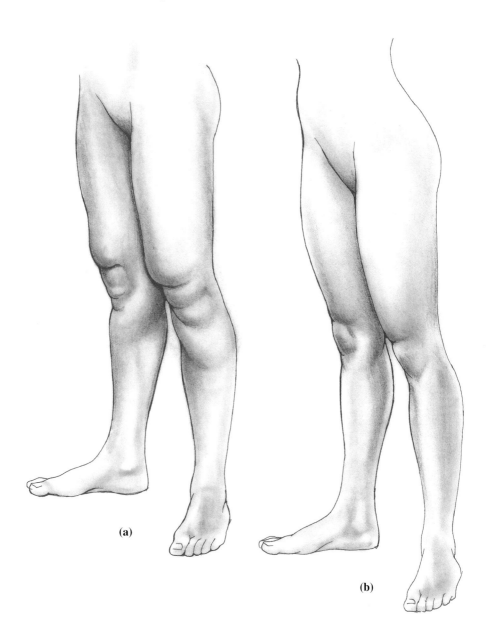

Figure 3-13. (a) Some women develop localized fat deposits on the inner aspect of the knees and also above the knee cap. **(b)** The contours can be improved with Tumescent Liposculpture.

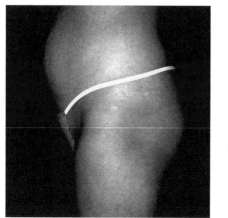 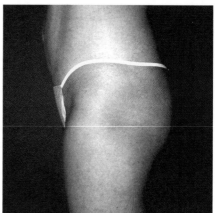

Used with permission, C. William Hanke, M.D.

Scheduling a Consultation

The first step for a person considering Tumescent Liposculpture is to consult a dermatologic surgeon who is experienced in the technique. "Old-style" liposuction is performed by physicians of different medical specialties and training, and experience varies widely. A surgeon should be chosen based upon his or her experience in Tumescent Liposculpture using tumescent local anesthesia, not just "old-style" liposuction under general anesthesia. Because liposuction has become so popular in recent years, many surgeons have added it to a long list of other procedures they perform. Few surgeons, however, are specifically trained and highly experienced in the science and art of Tumescent Liposculpture.

Tumescent Liposculpture is only performed with the specialized Tumescent local anesthesia in contrast to "old-style" liposuction which requires general or IV anesthesia. General anesthesia exposes patients to risks which are not found with local anesthesia. It is not necessary for a patient to undergo general anesthesia, hospitalization, and possibly blood transfusions to have unwanted fat removed. Tumescent Liposculpture is the safest and most comfortable method and is performed in the office surgery suite.

An interested patient can locate a dermatologic surgeon who is trained in Tumescent Liposculpture by calling the American Society for Dermatologic Surgery, 5550 Meadowbrook Dr., Suite 120, Rolling Meadows, IL, 60008 (toll-free 1-800-441-2737), or visiting the website at www.aboutskinsurgery.org. A friend who has had Tumescent Liposculpture may also be able to recommend a qualified dermatologic surgeon.

Once a person has located a dermatologic surgeon who is experienced in performing Tumescent Liposculpture, a consultation should be scheduled. During a consultation it is important that all questions be answered. It is wise to prepare in advance by reading as much about Tumescent Liposculpture as possible and writing down any questions. These questions might include, but are not limited to:

- Does the surgeon perform true Tumescent Liposculpture under local anesthesia or does he use "old-style" liposuction under general or IV anesthesia?
- How many Tumescent Liposculpture procedures does the surgeon perform per week?
- How long has the surgeon been performing Tumescent Liposculpture?
- Are patient references available?
- Are before and after photographs available?
- Is the surgeon active in teaching other surgeons the Tumescent Liposculpture technique?
- Has the surgeon written articles for medical journals or done research on Tumescent Liposculpture?
- What can I expect in terms of results?
- Have patients experienced complications following Tumescent Liposculpture?
- How long will it take me to recover afterwards?
- When will I be able to return to work and resume exercising?

The consultation usually begins by taking a medical history and a physical examination of the areas which are to be treated. The chances for improvement should be discussed. The consultant should discuss the details of the Tumescent Liposculpture procedure as well as the usual postoperative course. Fees must also be discussed so exact costs are known. In addition to the surgeon's fee, there may also be expenses for postoperative compression garments, preoperative blood work, medications, and use of the surgical suite.

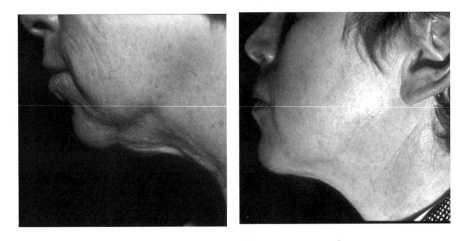

Used with permission, C. William Hanke, M.D.

The Tumescent Liposculpture Procedure

Preparing for Surgery

A decision to undergo cosmetic surgery should be made only after extensive research of the procedure and physician. A complete understanding of the postoperative course and anticipated outcome is essential.

Weeks Before Surgery

You should carefully plan for your surgery. The planning before, during, and after your procedure is important for a speedy recovery and maximum results.

Eat healthy foods

Begin your new healthy eating habits now. The best results are most often seen in patients who already have good eating habits or begin a diet and nutrition program prior to their Liposculpture procedure. Liposculpture can help you achieve the look you want, but you are ultimately responsible for what you eat. Even if patients have had trouble losing weight prior to surgery, it has been observed that after Liposculpture, most patients have an accelerated weight loss if they adhere to a program that includes reasonable exercise and a balanced low-fat diet. Please refer to Chapter 8 for precise information on nutrition.

Continue your exercise program

A firmer body means faster recovery and speedier results. Patients who have reasonable exercise programs in place before surgery, and continue them after surgery, achieve their final results more quickly than patients who do not exercise.

Discontinue certain drugs prior to surgery

You will be given a list of medications to discontinue prior to surgery. These may include, but are not limited to, aspirin and vitamin E (both slow blood clotting), anti-inflammatory medications, cold/flu medications (including over-the-counter cold remedies), ibuprofen (i.e., Motrin, Advil, etc.), herbs, and alcohol. These medications may increase your chance of bleeding during surgery. Ask the physician or nurse if your specific drug or vitamin is not on the list.

Smoking

Smoking is highly discouraged before and after any surgical procedure because it has been shown to slow the healing process.

Plan for your aftercare

Recovery with Tumescent Liposculpture is rapid and many people go back to work in one or two days. However, the immediate care after surgery is important for a comfortable recovery. You should plan to have a responsible person with you who will help you the first day and make sure you are eating properly and drinking the proper fluids. Most patients rely on family or friends. There are also numerous home-health care agencies that your physician can recommend. Your dermatologic surgeon can often provide a health care professional to stay with you the first night.

Most physicians prescribe medication prior to surgery. These usually consist of an antibiotic (to decrease the small chance of infection), and a mild pain medication for any postoperative discomfort. Most patients are comfortable taking only acetominophen (Tylenol). Make sure to get your prescriptions filled prior to surgery and start taking them as prescribed.

You will also be given a list of items that you may need to purchase for your postoperative care. Make sure you have these items on hand before your surgery. If you are having Tumescent Liposculpture of your face, be certain to have plenty of soft low-salt foods available. If you are having Tumescent Liposculpture of your body, you will need several absorbent briefs and/or pads or towels to absorb any excess anesthetic solution.

The Day of Surgery

Shower and wash your hair the morning of surgery. You may be given a special soap to use. Do not apply moisturizers or deodorant. Eat a light meal the morning of surgery. Do not consume caffeine.

Someone should drive you to the office surgical suite the day of your procedure. Even though you may only have a local anesthetic, you should not drive yourself home. Wear loose, comfortable, washable pants and shoes that can be removed easily. Wear a washable shirt or blouse that buttons or snaps so that you will not need to pull it over your head.

The nursing personnel will take you into the surgical suite to prepare you for your procedure. The surgeon will review with you the areas which he plans to treat, then mark those areas with a special skin marker. You may be given a medication to relax you either by mouth or injection.

In the office surgical suite, a special Tumescent solution will be infiltrated with a small cannula into the areas to be sculpted. The Tumescent anesthetic solution consists of very dilute lidocaine (a local anesthetic), very dilute adrenalin (to constrict blood vessels), sodium bicarbonate (to allow comfort during infiltration) and normal saline. During this phase of the procedure, most patients report that the skin feels stretched as if they had eaten too much. Most patients listen to music or chat with the nursing personnel during this part of the procedure; some talk on the phone or sing to the music. Once the infiltration process is complete, the areas to be sculpted have been completely anesthetized. You are relaxed and feel little or no discomfort. The surgeon then checks to see if all the areas are sufficiently anesthetized. You are now ready for the actual sculpting process.

The surgeon begins sculpting each area, using small cannulas of different lengths to achieve the best results. The surgeon gently pushes the Liposculpture cannula back and forth within the fatty tissue to remove the excess fat. This delicate process appears similar to a person playing the violin. The cannula is attached by clear tubing to a suction machine. The machine draws the fat into a container. During Tumescent Liposculpture, the suctioned fat is usually quite yellow because of the absence of bleeding. Once the sculpting is completed, the incisions are usually left open to allow the solution to drain from the sites, but some sites may be sutured. The advantage of leaving the incisions open is faster drainage of the solution, resulting in quicker recovery and less swelling. These tiny incision sites are usually only one eighth of an inch long and almost disappear after the surgery.

The actual sculpting can take from one to four hours, depending on the number of fatty areas and their size. The procedure takes time because the dermatologic surgeon sculpts your body much like an artist does. Patients appreciate the extra time that is spent giving the body a smoother contour. A surgeon trained in Tumescent Liposculpture will blend the areas to create a natural contour for your new figure. Tumescent Liposculpture is not a rapidly

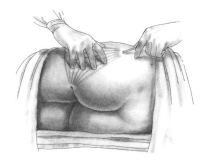

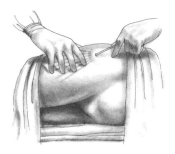

Figure 5-1. Tiny tunnels of subcutaneous fat are removed almost bloodlessly using Tumescent Liposculpture.

performed procedure. The experienced surgeon uses great patience to assure that each area is naturally contoured and symmetrical, and that the optimal amount of fat is removed.

After Surgery

Drink plenty of fluids. Be sure to eat normal meals..

Although much of the remaining Tumescent fluid is absorbed, some of the fluid drains out through the incision sites for several hours after the procedure. The fluid is collected on absorbent pads placed over the incisions. Special comfortable support garments are worn postoperatively to collapse the small tunnels in the fat. The small tunnels in the fat are compressed and gradually shrink in the weeks following Tumescent Liposculpture.

After Tumescent Liposculpture of the body, elastic shorts or girdles are usually used. Stretch waist bands or surgical binders also may be utilized. A special elastic head strap is used following Tumescent Liposculpture of the face and neck.

It is very important to wear the compression garment for the first two weeks after surgery to help contour the treated areas. These garments are light weight and can be worn in public without difficulty. Many patients continue to wear them for a portion of each day up to four weeks after their surgery.

Someone will need to drive you home. Plan for your driver to have sufficient time to go over your postoperative instructions with the doctor or nurse. Do not drive after surgery for the first 24 hours or longer if you are taking any pain medication.

Recovery from Tumescent Liposculpture is surprisingly rapid. Most patients spend the afternoon resting. The local anesthesia continues to be effective for the remainder of the day so very little, if any, pain medication is required. Some patients take a prescription medication for mild discomfort. Tylenol also may be used, but do not take aspirin or Motrin. Check with your physician before taking any medication.

Resume normal activity including showers after surgery, but do not sit in a bathtub, swim, or sit in a hot tub for three weeks or until the tiny incisions are completely healed.

You can move around easily the day after Tumescent Liposculpture and may resume normal activities. You may have tenderness that feels like you exercised too much the day before. By the second or third day most patients return to work without difficulty. Light exercise also can be resumed when you feel ready. Most patients comment that they undertake light exercise the day after surgery; many patients will walk two to three miles. Patients may resume their normal aerobic exercise program as soon as they desire following Tumescent Liposculpture.

Most patients are excited about their new shape following surgery, which will improve even more over the next few weeks as the swelling subsides. This swelling usually occurs immediately after the procedure and is normal. The body needs time to become adjusted to its new form. Most swelling can be diminished by wearing the compression garment or support stockings. Drinking plenty of fluids and resuming light exercise also are beneficial.

Some patients notice mild bruising in the areas that were sculpted. If you are the type to bruise easily, you may have more bruising after Tumescent Liposculpture than others who rarely bruise. Any bruises present usually fade quickly.

Most patients are back to their normal level of activity only days after surgery, already seeing a new improved figure. However, the final results of Tumescent Liposculpture continue to improve for six to 12 months. The benefits of Tumescent Liposculpture are dependent upon gradual tightening of the fatty layer and reduction of swelling. Exercise, proper diet, and plenty of fluids can speed your recovery, resulting in the figure you've always wanted.

Ultrasonic Liposuction

Specialized equipment using ultrasound technology is available for liposuction. In ultrasonic liposuction, a rapidly vibrating cannula is used to break up the fat before it is suctioned. This approach may be useful for liposuction of areas of the body which typically have very firm fat. These include the male flanks, male breasts, and the back.

However, ultrasonic liposuction has a number of drawbacks including larger scars and the potential for burns. Also ultrasonic devices take away much of the feel of the tissues for the surgeon and can lead to inadvertent penetration of deeper tissues. Most dermatologic surgeons no longer use ultrasonic liposuction.

External ultrasound may also be used. The ultrasound handpiece is rubbed over the area prior to Tumescent Liposculpture to break up the fat. The remainder of the Tumescent Liposculpture technique is the same.

Powered Liposuction

The latest breakthrough in liposuction technology is the use of powered cannulas to help remove fat. Powered liposuction devices feature a cannula which moves in an in and out direction about 3,000 times per minute. Powered liposuction has been shown to be more comfortable for patients than manual liposuction. Also powered liposuction appears to result in less trauma to the tissues resulting in less bruising and swelling. Many dermatologic surgeons prefer powered liposuction because these instruments make it physically easier for the surgeon to remove fat.

Can Fat That Has Been Removed be Used for Anything Else?

Patients frequently ask if fat removed from one area of the body can be used in another. Fat transplantation or fat transfer has been performed for many years with good results.

Fat has actually been transplanted from one part of the body to another for more than 100 years. However, until liposuction was developed, this involved literally cutting large portions of fat from one part of the body and placing it through a large incision in another part.

Tumescent Liposculpture allows physicians to suction fat with a small syringe and then immediately reimplant the material into another part of the body using only a needle. Individual fat cells are now being transplanted rather than a large block of fat.

Fat Transfer

Fat transfer is commonly utilized to correct loss of soft tissue in the face. One of the normal effects of aging is for fat to be lost in some areas while accumulating in others. For example, fat may be lost in the forehead, cheeks, chin, smile lines (between the nose and lips), and the lips themselves while accumulating in the jowls or along the jawline. Fat injections into the hollow areas serve to recontour the face. Many individuals with hollow cheeks who think they need a face-lift would be better served with fat transfer. In some people, fat may shrink with age, resulting in a "skeletal" or gaunt look. Fat transfer helps to replace this fat and can give a more natural, youthful appearance.

The percentage of fat which survives in its new location varies greatly from person to person. Most individuals will retain up to 40 percent of the transferred fat for long-term correction. Although living fat cells have been found many years after transplantation, it is not known whether the cells survive permanently. Patients usually require several procedures months to years after the initial transplantation to obtain the best results.

Fat can be transferred during Tumescent Liposculpture or as a separate procedure at another time. When it is performed separately, a small syringe attached to a small needle or cannula is used to harvest the fat from a body area. The procedure is performed using Tumescent local anesthesia. The fat can be injected immediately into the desired area. Minor bruising is common for a few days in both the donor site of the body and the treatment site. Extra fat can be harvested and stored in a freezer for injection at a later date. Recently, interest has developed in obtaining "autologous collagen" from suctioned fat cell walls which are broken down by ultrasound, freezing, and centrifugation.

Preliminary studies indicate that autologous collagen can produce a temporary correction for superficial wrinkles similar to that achieved with dermal fillers such as Zyderm, CosmoDerm, or Restylane. Fat transplantation, on the other hand, fills deeper and larger folds. The two methods can be used together to obtain a two-layer correction

Potential Complications

Any surgical procedure carries the risk of complications. The most serious complications of liposuction occur due to problems with general anesthesia used by some surgeons. Tumescent Liposculpture uses local anesthesia thereby minimizing the risks.

Excessive bleeding is a complication that can occur when "old-style" liposuction is performed without placing large amounts of the Tumescent anesthesia solution in the fat prior to the surgery. The Tumescent Liposculpture solution contains adrenalin that shrinks the blood vessels so they are less likely to bleed. When this special solution is injected into every portion of the fatty layer, there is minimal bleeding during the procedure.

In a small percentage of cases, blood clots have developed following "old-style" liposuction under general anesthesia. Research indicates that this complication is most likely to occur when liposuction is combined with other surgical procedures. This is especially true when it is performed at the same time as a "tummy tuck" or abdominoplasty. Consequently, most dermatologic surgeons recommend that Tumescent Liposculpture be performed as a single procedure and not at the same time as another surgery.

Infection is possible after any surgical procedure. For this reason, dermatologic surgeons have recommended that Tumescent Liposculpture be performed using a sterile technique. Furthermore, the *Clinical Guidelines for Liposuction* published by the American Academy of Dermatology endorse the use of antibiotics before, during, and immediately after the procedure in order to prevent infection. Infection following Tumescent Liposculpture is extremely rare.

In addition, there are a number of minor problems that may occur after the procedure. These are not dangerous to the health of the patient, but may be annoying. They include, but are not limited to, minor skin surface irregularities, temporary numbness, bruising, itching, sensitivity of the operative site, and tiny scars at the site of the cannula insertion.

A strong safety record has been achieved with Tumescent Liposculpture. In 1995, a National Survey of 15,336 patients who had undergone Tumescent Liposculpture was reported in the medical journal *Dermatologic Surgery.* (Hanke CW, Bernstein G, Bullock S. "Safety of Tumescent Liposuction in 15,336 patients." *Dermatol Surg* 1995;21:459, 459-462.) Sixty-six dermatologic surgeons contributed data on 44,014 body areas in 15,336 patients. There were no admissions to the hospital for treatment of complications and no blood transfusions in any of the patients. The complications that were reported were minor and infrequent.

In 2002, an additional national survey reported on 66,370 tumescent liposculpture procedures performed between 1994 and 2000. (Houseman et al, The safety of liposuction: results of a national survey. Dermatol Surg 2002; 28:971-978). The study reported no fatalities and a very low rate of complications.

What should you do next?

After reviewing the details of the Tumescent Liposculpture procedure in Chapter Five, the next step is to set up a consultation with a qualified doctor.

To locate a dermatologic surgeon near you, call the American Society for Dermatologic Surgery, 5550 Meadowbrook Dr., Suite 120, Rolling Meadows, IL. 60008 (toll-free 1-800-441-2737). www.aboutskinsurgery.org

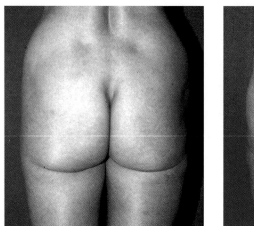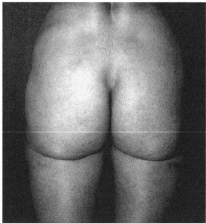

Used with permission, C. William Hanke, M.D.

Frequently Asked Questions About Tumescent Liposculpture

The following questions are frequently asked regarding Tumescent Liposculpture. The answers provided are general ones. More specific answers are tailored to the patients' needs and can be answered at a consultation.

Q. *What is the purpose of Tumescent Liposculpture?*

A. We are all victims of our own heredity. As we age we tend to develop hereditary areas of localized body fat that do not respond to diet and exercise. The common problem areas in women include the lower abdomen, upper outer thighs, upper inner thighs, hips, waist, buttocks, inner knees, arms and neck. The common problem areas in men include upper abdomen, lower abdomen, waist (love-handles), breasts, and neck. Tumescent Liposculpture allows correction of these problem areas safely and effectively under local anesthesia.

Q. *How safe is Tumescent Liposculpture?*

A. Tumescent Liposculpture is the safest method of liposuction available. In 1995, the American Society for Dermatologic Surgery published national survey data on 15,336 patients who had undergone Tumescent Liposculpture. The study was reported in the medical journal *Dermatologic Surgery* (Hanke CW, Bernstein G, Bullock, S, "Safety of Tumescent Liposuction in 15,336 patients." *Dermatol Surg* 1995; 21:459-462). The study reported no admissions to the hospital for treatment of complications and no blood transfusions in any of the patients. The complications that were reported were minor and infrequent. An additional study involving

66,370 patients was published in 2002 (Houseman et al. The safety of liposuction: results of a national survey. Dermatol Surg 2202; 28: 971-978). No fatalities were reported and complications were infrequent. In conclusion, Tumescent Liposculpture has a strong safety record.

Q. Will I need pre-operative blood tests and a physical exam?

A. Yes.

Q. Will I have pain?

A. There is minimal, if any, discomfort during administration of the Tumescent local anesthesia. Patients usually listen to music or talk with the nursing personnel during this time. During the Liposculpture procedure itself, the patient experiences virtually no pain. Many patients have compared the experience to a deep massage. The Tumescent local anesthesia keeps the patient comfortable for 18-24 hours after Tumescent Liposculpture. Mild oral pain medications are sometimes utilized for several days. Slight soreness of the surgical site is present for one to two weeks after Tumescent Liposculpture.

Q. Will I receive any sedatives?

A. Many patients prefer no oral sedation. Others prefer a mild oral sedative such as diazepam (Valium) or meperidine (Demerol).

Q. How many tiny incisions are necessary?

A. Generally two to twelve one-eighth inch incisions are required to treat a given body area. Most incisions are small and don't require sutures.

Q. What inconveniences can I expect following the procedure?

A. The Tumescent anesthetic fluid leaks from the tiny incisions for 18 hours following the procedure. This is a bother, but is only temporary.

Q. *What instructions will I receive before Tumescent Liposculpture?*

A. Written and oral instructions are provided in advance of the procedure.

Q. *How many days of work will I miss?*

A. Most patients return to work in two to three days. Many patients have Tumescent Liposculpture on Thursday or Friday and return to work on Monday.

Q. *What medicines will be prescribed for me after Tumescent Liposculpture?*

A. All patients receive pre-operative and post-operative antibiotics in order to minimize any chance for infection. All patients are given a prescription for a mild pain medicine, but less than half of them ever use it.

Q. *How soon after Tumescent Liposculpture can I take a shower?*

A. You may shower one day following Tumescent Liposculpture, but tub baths should be avoided for three weeks. Hot baths may increase swelling.

Q. *How long will I need to wear the compression garment?*

A. Patients wear a comfortable compression garment under their clothing 24 hours a day for the first week or two following Tumescent Liposculpture. They wear the garment for 12 hours a day for one or more additional weeks. Patients should not wear the garment beyond four weeks unless required by the physician.

Q. *Will I be bruised?*

A. Most people know how easily they bruise. Some patients have a tendency to bruise easily. Some patients have no visible bruising at all following Tumescent Liposculpture. If bruising occurs, it will resolve in two to three weeks. In general, bruising following Tumescent Liposculpture is minimal compared to "old-style" liposuction.

Q. What possible complications may occur?

A. The complications following Tumescent Liposculpture are minor and infrequent. Blood loss is minimal, so blood transfusions are unnecessary, unlike traditional liposuction under general anesthesia. A slight amount of bruising is common. Minor soreness of the treated area may last for several weeks. Infections and major complications are extremely rare. Occasionally skin irregularities may occur, especially in older patients who may have poor skin elasticity.

Q. When can I resume exercise?

A. Walking can be started on the day following surgery. Stretching and light weights may be used within a few days. Heavy aerobic type exercise should be avoided for 7-21 days depending on the body areas treated and the physician's advice.

Q. How long before sexual activities may be resumed?

A. Usually a day or two, but your body will tell you.

Q. How long will it be before I can see a noticeable improvement?

A. A small number of patients observe that their clothes fit more loosely within a few days. Many patients notice some improvement within one to four weeks. The final result is not apparent for six months or more.

Q. Will I have scars?

A. The tiny incisions are hidden in skin folds and other inconspicuous areas. They eventually become unnoticeable in most patients.

Q. What about alcohol consumption and smoking following Tumescent Liposculpture?

A. One drink per day probably will have no adverse effect after the first postoperative day. Smoking, of course, interferes with healing after any surgery.

Q. ***If I gain weight following Tumescent Liposculpture, will I gain in the areas that were treated?***

A.   The fat cells are permanently removed during Tumescent Liposculpture. Therefore, the treated areas can never become as large as they would have been if Tumescent Liposculpture had not been performed. However if you gain weight the fat may store elsewhere. Therefore you should maintain your current weight or better yet loose weight after liposuction.

Q. ***How much will the procedure cost?***

A.   The cost for Tumescent Liposculpture will vary depending upon the body areas treated, the time involved, and the experience of the physician. Your dermatologic surgeon can give you precise costs after examining you.

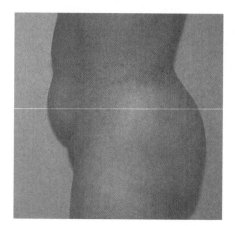 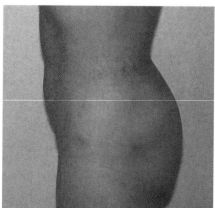

Used with permission, William P. Coleman III, M.D.

Definition of Terms

Banana roll - a roll of fat that sometimes develops on the back of the thigh just beneath the buttocks.

Cannula - a narrow tube that is used to suction fat from underneath the skin.

Cellulite - skin surface irregularities that arise from compartmentilization of the underlying fat.

Compression garment - a special garment that is worn for two to four weeks after Tumescent Liposculpture in order to collapse the fat tunnels and shape the new area.

Criss-cross liposuction - a criss-cross pattern that is made in the fat with small cannulas in order to remove fat evenly.

Dermatologic cosmetic surgeon - a dermatologist who has training and experience in surgery of the skin and adjacent tissues. Many surgical procedures have been developed or refined by dermatologic surgeons including hair transplantation, dermabrasion, chemical peel, sclerotherapy, cutaneous laser surgery, Botox injections, Mohs micrographic surgery for skin cancer, treatment of aging skin, and Tumescent Liposculpture.

Face lift (traditional) - an extensive surgical procedure that involves cutting out excess skin at the sides of the face and neck. A face-lift can sometimes be avoided or delayed by performing Tumescent Liposculpture of the neck.

Fat cells - body cells that are filled with fat. These cells swell and shrink as a person gains and loses weight.

Fat transfer - living fat cells are harvested from one area of the body and are transferred to another area (eg. lips) to add youthful fullness.

General anesthesia - a form of total body anesthesia that is given by face mask or endotracheal tube. General anesthetic agents cause vasodilation (i.e., widening of blood vessels) which increases bleeding. General anesthesia involves a recovery period that can include nausea and vomiting.

Generalized obesity - individuals with this condition are 20 percent or more over the recommended body weight.

Intravenous anesthesia - a form of deep sedation with risks similar to general anesthesia.

Jowl - an unattractive bulge of fat that hangs down from the jawline below the corner of the mouth.

Liposculpture - an advanced type of liposuction with sculpting of the body instead of just removing fat.

Liposuction - a method of removing excess body fat using suction.

Local anesthetic - an anesthetic agent that is injected into a localized area of soft tissue in order to anesthetize it.

Localized hereditary body fat - excess fat in "problem areas" which are inherited and depend upon the sex of the patient. They do not respond to diet and exercise. Common "problem areas" in men include the neck, abdomen, waist/love handles, and breasts. Common areas in women include the abdomen, inner and outer thighs, hips, waist, buttocks, inner knees, neck and calves/ankles.

Love handles - hereditary fat accumulations around the waist in men.

Microliposculpture - the art of using small, fine cannulas with great precision to remove fat in a more controlled fashion.

Obesity - a condition characterized by the accumulation of excessive amounts of body fat.

"Old-style" liposuction - this type of liposuction is performed under general anesthesia or intravenous anesthesia without the advantage of Tumescent local anesthesia. Following "old-style" liposuction, blood transfusions may be necessary to replace the blood that is suctioned along with the fat.

Pinch test - the skin and underlying fat are pinched between the thumb and index finger in order to measure the thickness. This test can help determine if Liposculpture is indicated.

Powered liposuction - a method for performing liposuction which utilizes a motorized cannula which rapidly moves back and forth dislodging fat cells in the process.

Saddle bags - excessive hereditary fat that accumulates on the outside of the thighs in some women.

Sedative - an oral medication such as Valium that is sometimes given to relax the patient before Tumescent Liposculpture.

Tumescent local anesthesia - the subcutaneous fat layer is anesthetized and made firm by injecting large volumes of a dilute mixture of lidocaine ("the anesthetic agent") and epinephrine (which constricts the blood vessels).

Tumescent Liposculpture - a new, safe, essentially painless method of liposuction that is performed entirely under local anesthesia. Blood loss is minimized which eliminates the necessity of blood transfusions.

Tummy tuck - an extensive surgical procedure that is performed under general anesthesia to repair abdominal muscles and remove fat. A long scar results. Tumescent Liposculpture can often eliminate the necessity of a "tummy tuck."

Turkey neck - excess fat accumulation in the neck with age causing multiple folds and a "double chin."

Ultrasonic Liposuction - a controversial method of liposuction which utilizes a rapidly vibrating cannula to assist in breaking up the fat.

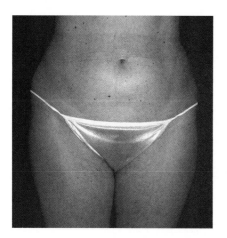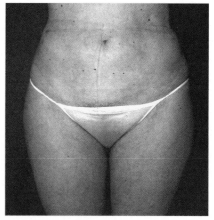

Used with permission, C. William Hanke, M.D.

Nutrition: Ten Techniques to Nourish Your Body for Wellness

Becky K. Zimmerman, R.D.

Michael F. Busk, M.D., M.P.H.

Sarah P. Hanke, B.S.N., R.N., R.D.

"This food is good for you, that food is bad for you, this food is too high in fat, that food is low in fat but has too much sodium and sugar." These statements about food are all too familiar to the dieter and weight conscious consumer. Information is plentiful about the perfect diet or food that will give you a model figure, improve your health, or prolong your life. All this information can be a bit overwhelming, not to mention confusing. However, as confusing as things seem, it's easier than you think to eat well without being compulsive and restrictive about food selections. The following are 10 techniques you can use to eat well and get the health enhancing benefits found in a variety of foods.

1. Be free of diets, eat for wellness.

Diets place restrictions on the types and amounts of foods you eat, and take the enjoyment out of feeding and nourishing your body. Diets are seen as a punishment used to correct something that is wrong with your body, and often end in disappointment and "failure." Food is the enemy for fearful dieters and certain foods are designated as "good" and "bad." If dieters eat a "good" food they are good people, if they eat a "bad" food, they are bad people. Diets generally dictate a specified amount of food to be eaten at a specified time regardless of the feelings of the presence or lack of physical hunger. Because most diets call for restricting caloric intake and eliminating certain foods, they may be nutritionally inadequate. A diet that recommends less than 1,200 calories per day is marginally adequate in many nutrients and should not be used for a long period of time.

It is common for people who lose weight on a diet to gain it back when they resume their old eating habits. This phenomenon (known as "weight cycling" or "yo-yo dieting") actually makes weight management more difficult for the long term. Each time a new diet is started a person loses both fatty tissue and lean muscle. This decrease in lean body mass actually slows the metabolic rate. A weight plateau is eventually reached that can be discouraging and may cause the dieter to return to old eating habits. When old habits return, fatty tissue also returns. This fatty tissue does not burn as many calories as lean tissue, which results in weight gain and another diet. Lifestyle change is the only effective way to lose weight and keep it off. Healthy eating without deprivation is the only way to keep your taste buds happy. Foods that are considered "bad" can still be enjoyed occasionally and in moderation.

Living without dieting allows you to enjoy and savor the taste of food. Food becomes much more satisfying because you choose what and when you want to eat. The desire for "forbidden" and "bad" foods diminishes because there are no forbidden foods. The results of eating for wellness is a well nourished body that gradually arrives at a healthy and natural body weight. Without dieting you are allowed to eat when you are physically hungry and stop eating when your hunger is satisfied.

Pearl: Consume at least 1,200 calories a day and choose a variety of foods. Stop letting diets control you. Regain the freedom of choosing to eat the foods you enjoy. Allow yourself the experience of pleasurable, guilt-free eating occasionally. If you allow yourself to have foods you enjoy you are less likely to binge on these foods at a later time. You will feel better mentally and physically. You will remove the barriers to the enjoyment of eating and eliminate the feelings of deprivation.

2. Use the pyramid principle and experience a variety of foods.

Use the pyramid principle to get a balance of foods daily. The Food Guide Pyramid is an estimation of daily needs that can be used as a guideline for healthy eating. Each food group offers a range of recommended number of servings in order to be useful to people of various sizes. For instance, someone needing fewer calories daily should consume a number of servings at the lower end of each range. A person needing more calories daily should consume a number of servings at the higher end of the range. Eating well, by using the Food Guide Pyramid to choose a variety of foods, can be interesting as well as healthy. It ensures that your body gets all the essential nutrients it needs to function normally. There is no single food or food group that contains all the nutrients your body needs. Let's take a look at what the pyramid has to offer.

At the base of the Food Guide Pyramid are energy packed grain foods, which provide B vitamins, iron (whole grains and fortified), and fiber. Choose whole grain breads, cereals, and various grains such as couscous, bulgur wheat, and brown rice for variety. One slice of bread or one-half cup of cooked rice or pasta provides you with one serving.

On the second level, the pyramid promotes an abundance of fruits and vegetables. These foods are abundant in the antioxidants beta-carotene and Vitamin C, and in phytochemicals all three of which may be helpful in the prevention of many diseases associated with aging, including cancer and heart disease. Fruits and vegetables are also rich in fiber and provide an additional source of fluid to our diet. The National Cancer Institute suggests we get at least five servings a day for good health. A serving is equal to one small piece of fruit, one-half cup cooked vegetables, or six ounces of juice.

On the third level of the pyramid the dairy and meat/protein foods are represented. Dairy foods are the major source of bone enriching calcium in the American diet. They also contain Vitamin D, riboflavin, and are a good source of protein. Choose low-fat (I percent, one-half percent, or skim) milk, yogurt, and cheese to reap the nutritional benefits provided by these foods. One serving is equal to one cup of milk or yogurt, or one and one-half ounce of cheese.

The meat/protein foods provide a variety of nutrients depending on what is chosen. Meats, poultry, and fish provide protein, iron, zinc, and some B vitamins. One serving of meat is two to three ounces, not the average 10 ounces Americans eat.

Pearl: Check yourself to see if you are getting at least the minimum number of recommended servings each day from the Food Guide Pyramid. The minimum number of servings includes six grains (three of these should be whole grains), a total of five fruits and vegetables, two servings from the dairy group, and two servings from the meat/protein group. Package labels do not always correspond with the serving sizes suggested by the pyramid, therefore it is important to learn to read labels. See the Food Guide Pyramid at the end of this chapter for information on serving sizes. Remember, enjoy new foods and recipes and stay out of an eating rut.

3. Choose an eating plan based on generous amounts of fruits, vegetables, whole grains, beans and legumes.

Consuming a "plant-based" diet plentiful in fruits, vegetables, whole grains, beans and legumes allows you to enjoy the many health protective characteristics present in those foods. Plant foods are naturally high in beta-carotene, Vitamins C and E (all antioxidants), soluble and insoluble fiber, and phytochemicals. They are naturally low in fat, saturated fat, cholesterol, sodium and sugar, and are low to moderate in calories, the excess of which contributes to ill health. Beans and legumes are free of saturated fat and cholesterol and are an excellent source of protein. They make a healthful and nutritious alternative to meat.

Pearl: Plan meals based on vegetables, grains, and legumes such as stir fry or casseroles, and add small amounts of meat or dairy foods to compliment the plant foods in the dish. Incorporate at least two non-meat meals per week into your eating plan. Here's an easy one that takes just minutes to prepare: Mix a can of red beans (rinse first) with cooked rice (use quick cooking) and season with chili powder, cumin, and pepper. Sprinkle on some grated low-fat cheddar cheese and serve with a tossed salad and fruit. It's a meal in minutes!!

4. Choose an eating plan that uses only small amounts of meat and whole milk dairy foods.

Meat and dairy foods can be a part of a healthy diet, but can contribute too much fat, saturated fat, cholesterol, and calories if used liberally in your eating plan. Minor adjustments (as suggested below) to decrease the amount of meat and high-fat dairy foods consumed will have a positive impact on your diet, and your food budget.

Pearl: To benefit from including these nutritious foods in your diet, choose lean meats (three to four ounces is a serving) and low-fat dairy foods (one to two ounces of cheese or a cup of milk per serving). When preparing casserole dishes containing meat and/or cheese, decrease the amount of these items and increase the grain or vegetables called for in the recipe.

5. Minimize your use of sugar, salt or sodium, caffeine, and alcoholic beverages, if you use them at all.

Processed foods containing added sugar and salt are generally lower in nutritional value than their unprocessed counterparts. Most foods containing added sugar provide little more than empty calories, lead to excess caloric intake, and weight gain. Consuming more than the recommended 2,400 mg of sodium per day, for some individuals, may contribute to hypertension.

Caffeine may cause nervousness and irritability in some individuals, and contribute to an irregular or rapid heartbeat. Consuming alcohol stimulates the appetite, which often leads to overeating in social settings where alcohol and food are found in combination. It is wise to eat before consuming any alcoholic beverages to slow the absorption of alcohol. Remember that alcohol provides extra calories that are of no nutritional value and may actually decrease the absorption of required nutrients from other foods.

The Food Guide Pyramid recommends a substantial reduction of total fat, saturated fat, and cholesterol. The Food Guide Pyramid is consistent with the 2000 United States Department of Agriculture (USDA) Dietary Guidelines for Americans and the 1996 American Cancer Society Guidelines on Diet, Nutrition, and Cancer Prevention. The pyramid indicates that healthful diets prevent excessive caloric intake by limiting the "empty" calories found in alcohol, caffeine, simple sugars, and salt. In addition to a healthful diet, eliminating smoking and increasing physical activity can decrease many risks of chronic heart disease and cancer.

Pearl: When choosing fruits and vegetables, choose fresh or frozen. Read the labels to be sure they have no added sugar or salt. Find other ways to flavor food without adding salt or sugar to cooked foods. Avoid instant or quick cooking foods because these foods are high in sodium. Limit your intake of beverages containing caffeine to one or two a day and to before noon. Moderate your intake of alcoholic beverages to no more than one or two a day, and don't drink on an empty stomach.

6. Avoid supplements and other gimmicks that make unrealistic claims or promises.

There is a wide array of dietary supplements available to the public. A dietary supplement is any vitamin, mineral, herb, or botanical that is intended for digestion that cannot be classified as a conventional food. Dietary supplements are not regulated in the same manner as food. Some supplements may actually be harmful if taken in excess, therefore it is important that the consumer has researched the supplement and discussed it with his/her physician. Dietary supplements are acceptable for people with certain health conditions (i.e. anemia, osteoporosis) or those who don't meet their nutritional requirements through their diet (i.e. vegetarians, or pregnant women).

There are many products available to the public that make unrealistic promises or have no scientific evidence to substantiate claims made on the packaging. Although all manufacturers should abide by the established guidelines, many do not. Consumers should be aware of deceptive marketing tactics including testimonials or unavailable research. In recent years there has been an increase in the availability of supplements that promise to boost metabolism and burn fat and help you lose weight. There is currently no research available to support these claims. These supplements may contain ingredients such as caffeine or ephedrine, which may cause tachycardia, hypertension, or palpitations. Any supplement should be used with extreme caution and under the supervision of a physician.

Pearl: Keep in mind that if a dietary supplement promises a quick fix or seems too good to be true — it probably is.

7. Eat to fuel your activities and lifestyle, don't skip meals through the day.

You can't expect to feel energetic in your daily activities if you don't fuel your body for those activities. Skipping meals and restricting your food intake results in an energy conserving body that slows down by lowering its metabolic rate and decreasing your desire for physical activity of any sort. Consuming meals and snacks throughout the day in response to your feelings of physical hunger is important in maintaining your energy level.

Eating throughout the day also keeps your mind sharper. Your brain requires a constant, steady, and generous supply of blood sugar to function properly. When you skip meals, your blood sugar level drops which results in a diminished supply of energy to the brain. This impairs your concentration, can cause headaches, irritability and fatigue.

Pearl: Eat regularly throughout the day. Choose a variety of foods from the pyramid to make balanced meals and snacks that satisfy your hunger.

8. Enjoy your foods in a slow and relaxed manner.

Stop to savor the flavor of the foods you are eating. You will derive much more enjoyment and satisfaction from your eating experience and be less likely to overeat. Eating on the run doesn't allow you to taste the foods you want to enjoy because you are focused on the activity or destination. Eating on the run is generally associated with hasty, less nutritious food choices and eating quickly. Maintaining a gentle awareness, without being compulsive, about your food choices allows you to eat healthfully and still enjoy eating. You simply cannot consume an abundance of fast foods, convenience foods, candy, cookies and other sweets and expect to not suffer some negative health consequences.

Remember, it takes at least 20 minutes for your stomach to signal your brain that it has had enough. If you eat quickly, by the end of 20 minutes, you may have consumed more calories than your body needed to satisfy its nutritional requirements and physical hunger. Eating in a hurried manner has a negative effect on digestion and absorption of foods as well. Eating on the run places other physical demands on the body that compete with digestion and absorption so you may not get the maximum nutrition from the foods you are consuming.

Eating is an activity we often take for granted and place low on our list of priorities. Lack of awareness, translates into poor health outcomes for most individuals. Take the time to plan a few healthy, great-tasting meals for you and your family. There are many excellent resources available to you for good and healthy family recipes. They are listed at the end of this chapter.

Pearl: In our fast paced lifestyles, slowing down to eat may be the only time we take in our day to relax. Make eating a calm and relaxing experience for you and your family.

9. Don't forget about hydration!

While food is important to nourish our bodies, me must not forget about the importance of remaining properly hydrated. An adult's body is composed of 55 to 75 percent water. Water regulates the body's temperature, transports nutrients and oxygen to your body cells and carries waste products away.

Most people need 8 to 12 cups of water daily. If you are healthy your body is able to easily regulate fluids. You feel thirsty when you need water and when you have consumed enough your kidneys are able to eliminate any excess fluids.

Pearl: Beware of fluids containing added sugars or caffeine. Water is the best choice because it contains no extra calories, sodium, fat or cholesterol. Juice and milk are healthier choices than soft drinks and other sugar containing beverages.

10. Enjoy the flexibility of normal eating.

Realize that there is room for flexibility in eating. On some occasions you may eat a little too much (holiday family meal) and on some occasions you may not eat quite enough (during illness or when feeling tired). That is okay. Listen to your body's signals. Trust your body's natural gauges and allow them to work. If you tune into your body's physical signals for nutrition, it will take good care of itself. Tuning into your body allows you to get back in touch with your physical hunger.

Physical hunger is the body's response to not having been fed for several hours, and is a painful feeling. Any type of food that provides the body with needed energy may satisfy physical hunger. Sometimes we feed a hunger that we mistake for physical hunger. This is emotional hunger or appetite. Emotional hunger occurs when we relate any number of feelings to a food. Boredom, grief, depression, loneliness, and happiness are all feelings that may prompt our emotional hunger. Feeding an emotional hunger often leads to overeating. Appetite is the result of a pleasurable association with a particular food. To satisfy an appetite, we seek out the specific food we find pleasurable.

Pearl: Learn the difference between your physical hunger and emotional hunger or appetite. Then allow yourself to eat when you are physically hungry and stop eating when that hunger is satisfied.

Conclusion

In your daily life, there are many things to think about and responsibilities to tend to. Taking care of yourself by providing your body with the foods that satisfy it are important in keeping you healthy so you can continue to fulfill your responsibilities. Maintain a gentle awareness, choose a variety of foods, and allow yourself the enjoyment that should accompany eating without making the task too time consuming and turning it into an obsession. Eating well is eating simply. Eating well and staying active are the keys to achieving and maintaining a healthy body and weight.

THE FOOD GUIDE PYRAMID

The pyramid can be used as a guide to daily eating,
with recommended servings and examples
from each category of food.

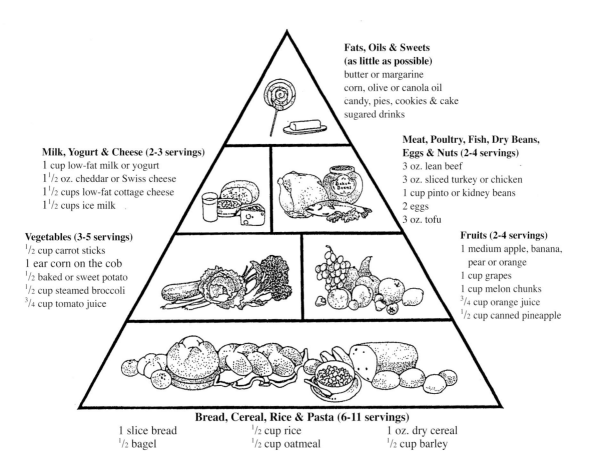

**Fats, Oils & Sweets
(as little as possible)**
butter or margarine
corn, olive or canola oil
candy, pies, cookies & cake
sugared drinks

Milk, Yogurt & Cheese (2-3 servings)
1 cup low-fat milk or yogurt
$1^1/_2$ oz. cheddar or Swiss cheese
$1^1/_2$ cups low-fat cottage cheese
$1^1/_2$ cups ice milk

**Meat, Poultry, Fish, Dry Beans,
Eggs & Nuts (2-4 servings)**
3 oz. lean beef
3 oz. sliced turkey or chicken
1 cup pinto or kidney beans
2 eggs
3 oz. tofu

Vegetables (3-5 servings)
$^1/_2$ cup carrot sticks
1 ear corn on the cob
$^1/_2$ baked or sweet potato
$^1/_2$ cup steamed broccoli
$^3/_4$ cup tomato juice

Fruits (2-4 servings)
1 medium apple, banana,
    pear or orange
1 cup grapes
1 cup melon chunks
$^3/_4$ cup orange juice
$^1/_2$ cup canned pineapple

Bread, Cereal, Rice & Pasta (6-11 servings)

1 slice bread	$^1/_2$ cup rice	1 oz. dry cereal
$^1/_2$ bagel	$^1/_2$ cup oatmeal	$^1/_2$ cup barley

PYRAMID MENU GUIDE

To help you with meal planning, you may use the MENU GUIDE along with the Food Guide Pyramid. By combining these tools you can select healthy foods in the proper amounts. Start with the first item listed in each meal and continue down the list choosing a variety of healthy foods. If serving size guidelines are followed this meal plan will provide you with approximately 1800 calories, 25% or fewer calories from fat, and 55% or more from carbohydrate not including snacks. Use the Food Guide Pyramid to determine appropriate serving sizes and food selections from each group.

MENU GUIDE

Breakfast
Fruit or Juice
Fiber-rich Cereal
Whole Grain Toast
Skim, $\frac{1}{2}$% or 1% milk
Margarine or Peanut Butter
Fruit Spread

Lunch
1 serving Protein (2-3 oz. lean meat or 1 cup legumes)
2-3 servings from Grains
2-3 servings from Vegetable and/or Fruit
Skim, $\frac{1}{2}$%, or 1% milk
Margarine, Salad Dressing, etc.

Dinner
1 serving Protein (2-3 oz. lean meat or 1 cup legumes)
2-3 servings from Grains
2 servings from Vegetable
Fruit or Light Dessert
Skim, $\frac{1}{2}$% , or 1% milk
Margarine, Salad Dressing, etc.

TIPS AND HINTS

1. Try to choose a vitamin C rich fruit or vegetable daily. This would include broccoli, cabbage greens, tomatoes, baked potatoes, cantaloupe, strawberries, oranges and grapefruit, and kiwi.

2. At least every other day choose a Vitamin A rich food. Foods include broccoli, carrots, greens, spinach, sweet potatoes, winter squash, apricots, cantaloupe, peach, pumpkin, and tangerine.

3. Try to limit your intake of added fats to a moderate 1-2 servings at a meal. One serving is equal to 1 teaspoon of regular margarine/butter, mayonnaise, or salad dressing. They generally contain about 45 calories and 5 grams of fat per teaspoon. Choose low-fat versions which have about half the calories and fat.

4. A light dessert might be a slice of Angel food cake, low-fat frozen yogurt, gelatin, ice milk, low-fat pudding, sherbet, sorbet, low-fat cookies or cakes. Remember, even though these foods are low-fat, they are often high in sugar and will provide too many calories if eaten in large amounts.

Snacks should be included in your daily meal plan as your activity needs allow. Choose healthy snacks to tide you over until meal time. Keep snack amounts small though so they don't become between meal meals!!

Prepared by Becky Zimmerman, RD
The National Institute for Fitness and Sport, 1995

On Your Way to Fitness:
Ten Steps to a Safe and Effective Exercise Program

Melanie A. Roberts, MS

Michael F. Busk, M.D., M.P.H.

Exercise can do many wonderful things for you. You may choose to exercise for a variety of reasons: to improve the functioning of your heart and lungs, to firm up your muscles and get stronger, to stay healthy longer, or to just feel better about yourself. As you can see, there is much more to being healthy than just looking good!

Whatever your reasons for exercise, it is important to follow some basic principles in order for your program to be safe and effective. In this chapter we will focus on 10 key steps to a successful exercise program.

1. Make a personal commitment to your health.

There is only one person who can keep you healthy — you. The habits you choose and the lifestyle you develop, whether good or bad, determines your health. Fortunately, most people have the choice of beginning an exercise program at will, on their own terms, when they are physically and mentally prepared to do so. Unfortunately, others wait until they are faced with what may have been a preventable disease, such as diabetes, obesity or heart disease, and a doctor says they must begin exercising to regain their health. The National Institute of Health (NIH) Consensus Development Panel indicates that these situations have become more common as 54 percent of adults in a 1991 survey engaged in either little or no regular leisure physical activity. Today, the Physical Activity and Health Report of the Surgeon General indicates that only 22 percent of adults engage in sustained physical activity of at least 30 minutes, five times a week. The same trend is occurring in today's children. The 1990 Youth Risk Behavior Survey indicated that the majority of high school teens did not regularly exercise, and that half did not participate in physical education classes. The Surgeon General reports daily attendance in high school physical education classes recently declined to 25 percent. Regular physical activity should be an integral part of maintaining health and fitness, throughout an entire lifespan.

As with any endeavor, your level of success in achieving health and fitness through exercise is related to your level of commitment. If you are already active, this may mean a more consistent workout schedule or perhaps fine tuning to an established routine. On the other hand, if you are just beginning to exercise, this means a commitment to a new lifestyle.

Whatever your task, don't think of exercise as a one-time immunization, but rather as a steady dose of preventive medicine that only works as long as it is administered. A few weeks (or even months) of regular exercise cannot erase years of inactivity and poor eating habits. Remember that exercise is the on-going process by which fitness and health improves, it is not an end in itself. Keep in mind as well that a good mixture of moderate and vigorous exercise training is beneficial (NIH Panel).

One of the best ways to begin your commitment and maintain your motivation is to find an exercise partner. This should be someone who has similar fitness goals and interests as yourself. It could be a neighbor, a friend, or someone you meet at a fitness center. When you use the buddy system you have someone who is counting on you to show up for a workout, and you are counting on them for encouragement. With the buddy system, you can both succeed in spite of each other.

So on your own or with a partner, make health your goal and use exercise as one of the paths to lead you there. With a strong commitment comes a strong sense of empowerment and control. And make no mistake about it, once you have the commitment, you can take control of your body...and take charge of your life. The NIH Panel stresses the importance of the positive mental attitude needed to successfully complete physical activity. An enjoyable activity allows for feelings of competency and safety in the activity, as well as minimizes negative consequences such as loss of time and injury. The Surgeon General's Physical Activity and Health Report indicates physical activity offers benefits such as reduced risk of coronary heart disease, hypertension, and premature mortality in general. Physical activity also offers improved muscle, bone, and joint health. Overall mental health may also be improved by reducing symptoms of depression and anxiety.

2. Notify your physician.

Anybody can exercise and you don't have to be a superstar athlete to enjoy the benefits of it. However, if exercise is new to you or if you change your current exercise program, it is important to inform your physician. Factors such as family history, your individual lifestyle, health status, and your age will influence the amount and type of exercise that is best for you. Based on your personal health history your physician may have important information regarding the parameters of your routine or perhaps exercises that you should avoid altogether. He or she may suggest a physical evaluation prior to beginning an exercise program. This is an ideal way to safely begin your program.

If you do not have a doctor, this is an excellent time to find one and to build a relationship with a professional that can provide you with general health care. Your doctor may also suggest that you meet with a fitness specialist who can develop an exercise prescription to meet your physical needs.

3. Set short and long term goals.

To have health and happiness is a vision. To reach the realm of reality it has to be identified as a goal — something with focus, something with an action plan. Begin your fitness program with a plan. Use a step-by-step process to set your fitness goals and turn your vision into reality.

Vision: Before you plan you must know what you want. You must also deeply believe it is possible before you can achieve it. Visualize yourself with the qualities of health and fitness that you will possess and the lifestyle you will have — once you've achieved your goal. Focus on your vision by writing down the most important reasons you have for wanting to achieve your fitness goal. *Example*: I will arrive at work refreshed and invigorated after I exercise in the mornings.

Mission Statement: Write down your specific long-range goal. Make it a simple statement of exactly what you want to accomplish by becoming more physically fit. This will help identify what you need to do to reach your goal. *Example*: I will reduce my body fat by 3 percent (which may equal six lbs.) over the next six months.

Action Plan: Break down your long-range goals into short-term, "working goals." Your working goals should specifically state the activity or behavioral changes you will implement. These are the roads you will take to success. Working goals should outline, in detail, the what, when, how much, and how often of your action plan. *Example*: I will begin with three days of exercise by either walking, jogging, biking or stair climbing for at least 30 minutes. Every two weeks I will add five minutes to my workout until I reach 45, maybe even 50 minutes of activity. I will ask a fitness specialist to design a weight lifting program so I will lift twice a week. I will eat two pieces of fruit a day and substitute fresh vegetables for any type of fried foods I may be tempted to eat.

Review and Assessment: Use each working goal as a check point to evaluate your progress and to implement changes when necessary. In many cases, flexibility is important. It allows you to adapt a new strategy if you realize that the steps you've been taking are ineffective, or it gives you the freedom to revise your time-frame if you find the first one too ambitious. *Example*: My exercise is going great, but I need to further improve my diet. I will meet with a dietitian and determine what I need to do to keep my daily fat intake below 25 percent of my total calories.

Reward: With the attainment of each working goal, plan to reward yourself for the accomplishment (no matter how small). Positive feedback will help small success breed greater success and continue to fuel your motivation. *Example*: I will buy myself something new to wear while exercising at the end of each month after I complete my working-goals.

4. Focus on the five essential components of physical fitness.

No single form of exercise is enough to develop and maintain optimal health and fitness. You should participate in a well-rounded health-promotion program that includes proper nutrition, good health habits, and exercises for strength, endurance, and flexibility. This not only provides you with variety, it also allows you to reach a higher level of total physical fitness. A complete fitness program is built on five essential components of physical fitness:

Cardiorespiratory Endurance (aerobic fitness): the optimal functioning of the heart, lungs and vascular system (blood vessels).

Muscular Strength: the maximal amount of force a muscle group can exert at one time.

Muscular Endurance: the capacity of a muscle group to continue physical performance over a period of time; to withstand fatigue.

Body Composition: the relative amounts of fat and lean tissue (muscle, bone and organs) in your body.

Flexibility: the range of motion around a joint.

If you are a member of a health-fitness facility you may have access to a variety of exercise equipment. If your are looking for such a facility, inquire about the qualifications of their staff. Make sure they have instructors with degrees in exercise science and certifications from professional organizations. A fitness instructor should be available to you while you are exercising, to answer questions and to assist you with your workout. Ideally, you will want to have a member of their professional staff assist you in designing a program that best fits your needs. Ask if they can provide you with a fitness assessment, whereby they test you in each fitness component, to take an objective measurement of where you are starting from. With this information an exercise prescription can be designed around your strengths and weaknesses and your progress can be charted over time.

If you do not wish to join a health-fitness facility, it is still worth the investment to hire a qualified personal trainer for a few sessions in order for him or her to provide you with a fitness assessment and an exercise prescription based on your present level of fitness and individual goals.

5. Develop your exercise program using the four fundamental factors of exercise.

Although your fitness program should be tailored to your individual goals and needs, the basic principles for a sound program are the same for all healthy adults.

There are four fundamental factors to consider when developing your total exercise program: (1) mode — type of exercise; (2) frequency of exercise

— how many exercise sessions per week; (3) duration — how many minutes of exercise and (4) intensity — how hard you are working.

Mode: type of exercise, such as walking, cycling, weight lifting.

The mode of your activity should vary from one session to another. This helps to not only combat overuse injuries, but also the mental boredom that can result from performing the same activities over and over. Keep in mind what activities you like for aerobic fitness and balance these either within your workout or on alternating days with resistance training exercises. This provides you with a well-rounded fitness program that is less likely to cause burn-out.

Frequency: how often you do the exercise.

Frequency, along with duration and intensity, affect the effectiveness of your exercise program. Although it is recommended that you complete three to five exercise sessions per week, do not exercise on a day when you feel that you have not sufficiently recovered from a previous exercise session. If you are too sore, too tired or feel local muscle fatigue, you may have over extended yourself in your previous session. In this case, you should allow your body enough recovery time in order to feel fresh and fully invigorated as you begin your exercise session.

Intensity: how hard you work.

Intensity is perhaps the most important factor in your program. Through exercise you are making your cardiovascular and muscular systems respond to an overload from which they become stronger and more efficient. With aerobic exercise, you measure this overload by taking your heart rate. With resistance training exercises, the overload can be measured by the amount of weight lifted or the number of times (repetitions) a weight is lifted.

Duration: **how many minutes you exercise.**

Each aerobic session should consist of 20-60 minutes of continuous activity. The duration of each session is directly related to the intensity of the activity and your present level of fitness. For example, activities at a lower intensity should be conducted for a longer period of time. Place emphasis on the total work you perform or on the total calories you burn. If you are beginning at a slow pace, it may be beneficial to keep track of how much work you are doing by recording how many miles you travel, either by walking, jogging, or cycling. For example, if you are just beginning to exercise and walking is your choice, walk for three miles rather than 30 minutes; regardless of your pace your calorie expenditure will be similar for that distance.

6. Learn to measure your heart rate.

A key ingredient in your exercise plan is your target heart rate (THR) zone. Heart rate refers to the number of beats your heart pumps in one minute. Since your heart has to pump oxygen rich blood to the working muscles in proportion to the workload, it pumps faster as the intensity of the exercise increases. This is a good way to measure the intensity of your aerobic exercises — by how many times your heart beats per minute (bpm).

Everybody has a resting heart rate (RHR) and a maximal heart rate (MHR), both of which are used to determine a THR zone. Your THR zone is a key factor in making significant progress in your fitness program. It represents a safe and reasonable intensity for most people while at the same time providing enough of an overload that the cardiovascular system becomes stronger and more efficient.

There is a simple formula to use for computing your THR zone. First, determine your RHR by taking your pulse immediately after waking up in the morning. Do this with your index and middle fingers at the carotid artery, which is located between the muscle along the side of your neck and your Adam's apple **(Fig. 9-1).** You can also take it at the radial artery running along the thumb-side of the front of your forearm **(Fig. 9-2).** Next, determine your predicted MHR by subtracting your age from 220. Plug these two figures into the following equations to find the upper and lower levels of your THR zone:

Formula for Estimating Your Target Heart Rate Zone

$$220 - \underline{\hspace{1.5cm}} = \underline{\hspace{1.5cm}} \text{ Maximal Heart Rate (MHR)}$$
Your Age

$$(\underline{\hspace{2cm}}) - (\underline{\hspace{2cm}}) = \underline{\hspace{3cm}}$$
Maximal HR   Resting HR   Heart Rate Reserve

$$(\underline{\hspace{2cm}}) \times 0.70 = (\underline{\hspace{1.5cm}}) + (\underline{\hspace{1.5cm}})$$
HR Reserve   Intensity Level   Resting HR

$$= \underline{\hspace{1.5cm}}$$
Target HR

Therefore, your target heart rate at 70% intensity = _____ (bpm)

Determine your target heart rate training zone by completing the above formula for the 50%-85% intensity levels:

Training Intensities as a Percent of Your Heart Rate Reserve

50% HRR = _____bpm	or	_____b/10 seconds
55% HRR = _____bpm	or	_____b/10 seconds
60% HRR = _____bpm	or	_____b/10 seconds
65% HRR = _____bpm	or	_____b/10 seconds
70% HRR = _____bpm	or	_____b/10 seconds
75% HRR = _____bpm	or	_____b/10 seconds
80% HRR = _____bpm	or	_____b/10 seconds
85% HRR = _____bpm	or	_____b/10 seconds

Now that you know your target heart rate zone, you can more carefully monitor your workouts. The best way to measure your heart rate is to check your pulse immediately after you stop exercising. At this time, the pulse beats will be rapid and strong; hence, easier to locate. Find your pulse within a second or two of stopping exercise and count for 10 seconds. Multiply this 10 second count by six to get your one minute heart rate.

The table below presents a chart for converting 10-second pulse counts to beats per minute. For example, 24 beats in 10 seconds is equivalent to a heart rate of 144 beats per minute.

TABLE 9-1. Conversion of 10-second pulse counts to beats per minute counts

10-Second Pulse Counts	Beats Per Minute Pulse Counts
15	90
16	96
17	102
18	108
19	114
20	120
21	126
22	132
23	138
24	144
25	150
26	156
27	162
28	168
29	174
30	180

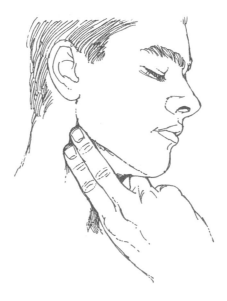

Figure 9-1. Carotid Pulse

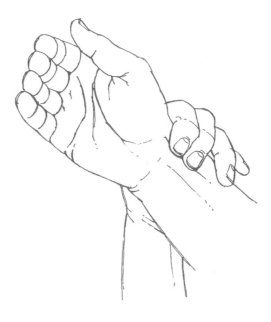

Figure 9-2. Radial Pulse

7. Begin your workout with a warm-up and finish with a cool-down.

The purpose of a warm-up is to prepare your body, especially your cardiovascular and musculoskeletal systems for the conditioning phase of your workout. Begin slowly and progressively increase the intensity of the exercise over a 10 minute period. It is best to use a form of exercise that closely mimics the type of exercise you are preparing for and involves similar muscle groups. Overall, the intensity should be 40-60% of your THR zone, and as a rule of thumb, your body is warmed-up once you break a sweat.

Just as the warm-up is used to prepare your body for exercise, the cool-down is used to allow your body to recover from exercise. The key is to allow your heart rate, blood pressure and body temperature to gradually return to resting values. You never want to suddenly stop moving or stand still while you are in the middle of an aerobic workout, when your heart rate is high. Because the contractions of your leg muscles are responsible for returning blood to your heart, a sudden cessation of activity causes a potentially dangerous pooling of blood in the lower extremities that can led to lightheadedness and dizziness. A thorough cool-down consists of 10-15 minutes of light, continuous activities (preferably similar to the previous heavier work) at a slower pace that does not cause your body to continue sweating.

8. Increase your cardiorespiratory capacity and improve your body composition with aerobic activities.

Cardiorespiratory capacity refers to the ability of your heart, lungs and blood vessels to take in and deliver oxygen to the working muscles. Being physically fit means having your heart, lungs, blood vessels and muscles functioning at peak efficiency. When you are in good physical shape you carry out your everyday activities with more energy and enthusiasm and activities such as long walks or hiking through the woods become simple pleasures.

Seen as one of the most essential components of physical fitness, aerobic fitness is reached through a program of aerobic exercise. Aerobic exercises are those activities that use large muscle groups, that can be maintained continuously and that are rhythmical and aerobic in nature. To be effective, however, aerobic exercises must be performed with sufficient frequency, intensity and duration to achieve your target heart rate training zone. Aerobic activities include:

* walking	* cross country skiing
* running	* rowing
* swimming	* aerobic exercise classes
* biking	* rope jumping

Aerobic exercise aids in the control of obesity, high blood pressure, high blood cholesterol, diabetes, and stress — all factors related to the development of cardiovascular disease. Body composition improvements result from both types of exercise — body fat is lowered by the extra calories burned through aerobic exercise and lean muscle is built in response to the resistance exercises.

FOR CARDIOVASCULAR ENDURANCE AND
IDEAL BODY COMPOSITION

Mode: Aerobic exercises — walking, jogging, cycling, stair climbing, aerobic exercise classes.

Frequency: 3 to 5 days per week.

Duration: 20-60 minutes per session.

Intensity: 40%-85% Training Heart Rate Zone

FORMAT

Warm-up: To prepare your body for exertion, begin your chosen activity slowly. Continue to work at a mild pace for about 10 minutes. As your body feels warm and your joints begin to loosen, gradually increase your intensity until you reach your desired training heart rate zone and continuing into the Training phase.

*If you feel any unusual muscle or joint stiffness during this warm-up, you should stop the activity and complete specific stretches for the area.

Training: *Initial Conditioning Stage*: This stage typically lasts the first 4-6 weeks, but may last longer depending on your previous level of fitness and your adaptation to the exercise program. Exercise at a level of intensity estimated between 40%-70% of your THR zone in order to avoid undue muscle soreness, injury, or discouragement.

Improvement Conditioning Stage: This stage lasts 12- 20 weeks, and is the period in which progression is the most rapid. Increase your intensity level to 50%- 85% of THR zone. Adapt your frequency and increased intensity levels by the rate at which you adapt to the conditioning program.

Maintenance Stage: When you have reached the desired level of conditioning, the maintenance stage begins. Now it is time to use your improved level of fitness to enjoy some of the more diverse lifetime activities.

Cool-down: A 5-10 minute cool-down period allows your muscles to assist in pumping the blood from the extremities back to the heart. Tapering off also allows your breathing and heart rate to return to near normal levels. After this gradual decline in activity is the perfect time to go through the stretching exercises outlined in step #10. The best time to focus on increasing joint flexibility is after a thorough cool-down.

9. Improve your muscle and bone strength with resistance training.

The resistance training exercises outlined here are designed to firm, shape, and contour muscles. Although these exercise won't result in spot reducing or massive losses in body weight, they will improve your girth measurements. These exercises emphasize body areas where most people typically experience a loss in strength and muscle tone: stomach or abdominal muscles, legs, buttocks, chest, back and arms. Although these exercises can firm and reshape your body for that fit look, they will not change your individual body type. For example, toning exercises cannot change a stocky, heavily muscled women into a thin or slender one. Nor should a women be afraid of becoming muscle-bound, women just do not have enough of the male-dominate hormone, testosterone, to develop large, bulky muscles. Besides, muscle toning is a slow process that allows you to train your body for the results you want.

The muscles that you develop are good for more than just looks. They are both the body's source of power and the key to a revved-up metabolism, the pace at which your body burns calories. As people become inactive (not necessarily older), they lose muscle, grow weaker, develop a sluggish metabolic rate and put on inches of fat even if they don't eat more. Dieting without resistance training can have the same effect — shedding muscle along with fat and ultimately slowing down the rate at which the body burns calories. Because resistance training stokes up the metabolic engine, building muscle mass is an efficient way to incinerate stubborn layers of fat. Though aerobic exercises burn calories during the activity itself, lean muscle mass consumes calories 24 hours a day, just to maintain itself. Pound for pound, muscle burns 40-50 more calories a day than fat burns. So putting on just three pounds of muscle will consume an extra 120 to 150 extra calories every 24 hours, even while you sleep.

As an added benefit, resistance training helps to decrease the likelihood of injuries by strengthening connective tissue and also aids in the prevention of osteoporosis by stimulating bone growth. As muscular fitness is being recognized as one of the cornerstones of independent living, we are discovering that many of the physical problems associated with aging are not chronological, but are actually the consequences of inactivity. Several studies show that nonexercising Americans lose at least 30 to 40 percent of their strength and 10 to 12 percent of their muscle mass by the time they are 65. This is hardly conducive to performing daily tasks — much less maintaining a fit and healthy body. Resistance training, as described by the NIH Panel, is essential for improving muscular function as well as potentially offering cardiovascular benefits. For people with Cardiovascular Disease (CDV) and older people, resistance training may be particularly enjoyable because of the potential for an increase in accomplishment of daily tasks. The Surgeon General's Physical Activity and Health Report also indicates that resistance training, when substituted for cardiorespiratory endurance activity at least twice per week for adults, helps maintain independence for the completion of daily activities. The improvements in musculoskeletal health also reduces the risks of falling at an elderly age. The good news is that it is never too late for a person (regardless of age) to stop, or even reverse muscle loss— here is how you can get started.

Developing Your Resistance Training Program
1. Select your exercises: incorporate all of your major muscle groups (legs, buttocks, chest, back, shoulders, arms and abdominals) into 8-10 exercises. Focus on the larger movements that work more than one muscle group at a time, such as the leg press, squat or lunge for the legs and the chest press, bent over row, and shoulder press for the chest, back and shoulders, respectively.

2. Order your exercises: begin your workout with exercises using the largest muscle groups first and work towards those using the smallest muscle groups last. Larger movements are designed to strengthen the largest muscle groups performing the movement. If you pre-fatigue a smaller muscle first, the larger muscles are not taxed and you compromised the possible gains from the exercise. For instance, if you start your workout with modified sit-ups, you'll fatigue your abdominal muscles — muscles that should be exercised last. This causes a problem when you move on to an exercise that relies on the abdominal muscles for support (such as the squat or shoulder press).

3. Determine your repetitions, sets and weight: these three variables measure the amount of work you do and in a big way, determine the results you get from your program. A repetition is performing a specific lift one time. A set is a group of repetitions performed together, without stopping. Three sets of 10 repetitions is recorded as three x 10. The amount of weight you use determines the training effect, whether it be muscle strength or endurance. Training programs that emphasize high resistance with few repetitions enhance gains in strength, muscle size, and to a lesser degree, endurance. Programs that emphasize a relatively low resistance with many repetitions enhance muscle endurance and, to a lesser degree, strength. This illustrates the degree to which resistance training can be controlled in order to achieve specific results — you can be the artist.

It is important not to use too much weight as you begin your program. The first three to four weeks should be devoted to learning the exercises. During this time the weight needs to be light enough that you can complete 10-12 repetitions with upper body exercises and 12-15 repetitions with lower body exercises. This is important so that you learn the movements and allow your nervous system to communicate with the muscular system in order to get the correct muscles to respond.

After this initial conditioning phase, gradually increase your resistance so that your muscles become fatigued within the given repetition range of your training objective — 6-8 reps for muscle strength or 12-15 reps for muscle endurance. As you become stronger you will be able to complete your sets at a given weight with relative ease. This is when you know it's time to add more resistance. If your goal is to complete 10 reps and you can get 11 or 12, then slightly increase your weight. You may only get six or eight reps on your next set, but stay with that weight until you can again complete 10 reps per set.

4. Determine your rest periods between sets: Between lifting sets you need to stretch the muscle groups you just worked. This is a great way to improve your flexibility. If you are training for muscle endurance you will want to have a rest period of about 60 seconds between lifting sets. For muscle strength this rest period is longer, 60-90 seconds, so that the nervous system has more time to recover, thus allowing you to lift heavier weights.

5. Determine how much time between workouts: Allow at least one full day between workouts using the same muscle groups. Because of time, you may choose to work your lower body one day and your upper body the next. Just make sure that you give your muscles enough time to recover. If your muscles feel tired or sore from a previous workout, then they have not had sufficient time to recover. You want to feel strong as you begin your workout.

FOR MUSCULAR STRENGTH AND ENDURANCE

Mode: Resistance machines

Free weights (barbells & dumbbells)

Body weight exercises (push-ups, sit-ups, chin-ups)

Frequency: Each major muscle group should be exercised a minimum of 2, but generally not more than 3 times per week; alternating days.

Duration: Each lifting set lasts approximately 30 seconds and has a 60-90 second recovery period between sets. A complete routine should take 20-45 minutes, depending on the number of exercises.

Intensity: For muscular endurance — fatigue between 12-15 repetitions; 2-4 sets per exercise.

For muscular strength — fatigue between 6-8 repetitions; 2-3 sets per exercise.

FORMAT

Warm-up: To prevent injuries, a proper warm-up is necessary. Range of motion exercises, as well as slow static stretches of the muscle groups to be worked are included in the warm-up session. Refer to the stretching guidelines in step #10.

Training: Exercises should be performed in a controlled manner. Maintain proper breathing during all lifts by exhaling during the exertion or lifting phase and inhaling during the recovery or lowering phase. Rest 60-90 seconds between sets. During this time, stretching of the muscle group being exercised is necessary.

Cool-down: If you do not begin your aerobic fitness workout immediately after your resistance training, a slow, static stretching routine is the perfect cool-down. The muscles are warm and will stretch much easier. This will help to not only increase flexibility, but will also decrease muscle soreness.

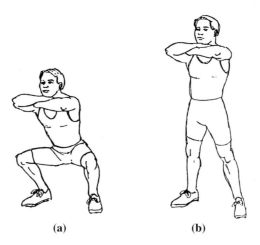

(a)   (b)

Figure 9-3. Freehand Squat

Muscles Used:	Quadriceps, Hamstrings, Gluteals
Starting Position:	Stand with your feet slightly more than shoulder width apart and your arms crossed in front of your chest.
Description:	Slowly lower your buttocks until the back of your thigh is parallel to the floor. Pause, then slowly return to the starting position.
Points to Emphasize:	•Keep your head up with eyes looking forward, back straight, and knees slightly out. •Inhale during the downward movement and exhale during the upward movement. •Do not bounce at the bottom of the movement. •Do not lock out your knees at the top of the movement. •Keep your weight on your heels, not your toes. If needed, use heel supports, such as a two x six piece of wood or a five pound weight plate, until your ankle flexibility increases. •As your strength increases, you may want to hold dumbbells in your hands.

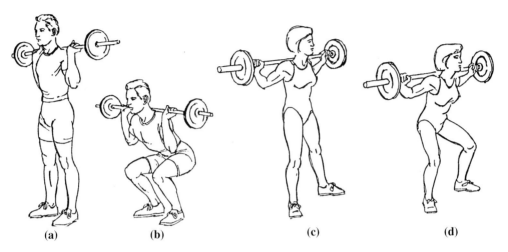

(a)   **(b)**   **(c)**   **(d)**

Figure 9-4. Barbell Squat

Muscles Used:	Quadriceps, Hamstrings, Gluteals, Spinal Erectors
Starting Position:	Stand with your feet slightly wider than shoulder width apart and the barbell resting on your shoulder and trapezius (upper back). Do not lock out your knees. Use a comfortable overhand grip.
Description:	Slowly lower your buttocks until the back of your thigh is parallel to the floor. Pause, then slowly return to the starting position.
Points to Emphasize:	•Keep your head up with eyes looking forward, back straight, and knees slightly out. •Inhale during the downward movement and exhale during the upward movement. •Do not bounce at the bottom of the movement. •Keep your weight on your heels, not your toes. If needed, use heel supports, such as a two x four piece of wood or a five pound weight plate, until your ankle flexibility increases. •Always use spotters or a safety rack when performing this exercise (not shown in diagram). •If you find it uncomfortable to rest the barbell across your shoulders, hold a dumbbell in each hand instead.

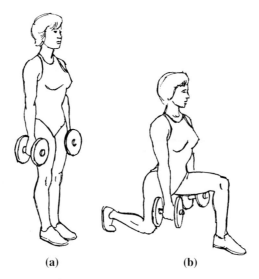

(a)   (b)

Figure 9-5. Dumbbell Lunge

Muscles Used:	Quadriceps, Gluteals, Hamstrings
Starting Position:	With your feet comfortably together, stand with your arms down at your sides, holding a dumbbell in each hand.
Description:	Stride forward with one leg. Slowly lower your body so that your front thigh is parallel to the ground and your trail leg is extended behind you. Your back knee should be lowered two to three inches above the floor. Push back with your front leg, keeping your trunk erect. Pause, then slowly recover to the starting position. Alternate legs. Try to push your body back to the starting position with one drive from your front leg.
Points to Emphasize:	•Learn this movement without dumbbells, using only your bodyweight and gradually increase the resistance.
	•Keep your trunk erect.
	•Inhale as you step out and exhale as you push off the front leg to return to the starting position.
	•Keep front knee directly over front foot as you lower your body weight. Never allow your front knee to travel forward over your toes. Your front knee should be bent at 90 degrees as you lower your body weight.

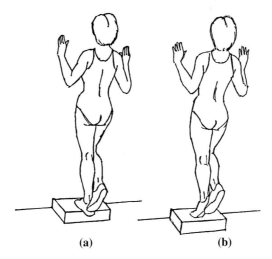

(a)   (b)

Figure 9-6. Heel Raise

Muscles Used:	Gastrocnemius (calves)
Starting Position:	Stand with your toes on a piece of wood, a barbell plate, or on a step. Balance yourself by placing hands against wall or handrail. Place left foot against right heel.
Description:	Raise up on toes as high as possible. Hold position momentarily and return to starting position, with heel dropped below toes as far as possible. Immediately raise your heels again allowing no time for rest or recovery. After completing desired number of reps, reverse position and repeat movement with left leg.
Points to Emphasize:	•In the starting position, place your toes in a position higher than your heels.
	•Keep your back straight, head up and knees locked.
	•Do not move hips backward or forward.
	•Do not bounce or move your knees as you do this exercise.
	•You can increase your resistance by holding a dumbbell in one hand.

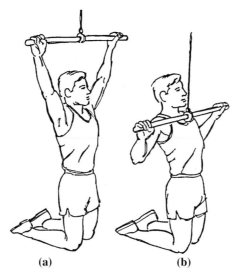

(a)   (b)

Figure 9-7. Lat Pull Down (on machine)

Muscles Used: Latissimus dorsi, biceps

Starting Position: Facing the weight stack, grasp the handlebar with an overhand grip wider than shoulder width. Kneel or sit down far enough to support weights with arms extended overhead.

Description: Pull the bar straight down until it touches your upper chest. Pause, then slowly return to the starting position and repeat.

Points to Emphasize: •As you pull the bar down concentrate on pulling your elbows behind you by using your back muscles.
                      •Exhale through the downward movement, inhale during the upward movement.
                      •An underhand grip, that is slightly narrower, may be used to place more emphasize on the biceps muscle.

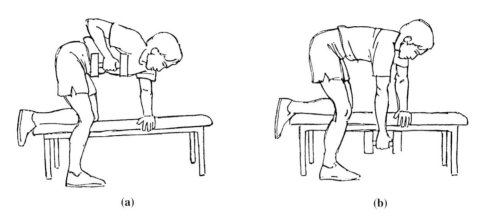

(a)   (b)

Figure 9-8. Dumbbell Bent-over Row

Muscles Used:	Latissimus dorsi, biceps
Starting Position:	Stand at one side of the bench. Kneel on the bench with your inside leg. Lean forward and place your inside hand on the bench 12-18 inches in front of your knee. Plant outside foot at side of bench and slightly bend knee. Position torso parallel to the floor, with back flat and stomach held in. Grasp dumbbell with outside hand. Hang dumbbell with elbow fully extended.
Description:	Pull dumbbell up, even with chest. Keep upper arm and elbow next to ribs. Keep back and shoulders even and parallel to floor. Touch dumbbell to outer chest and rib cage, then slowly lower dumbbell to the starting position and repeat. Reverse position and repeat movement on opposite side.
Points to Emphasize:	•Keep your head up, your back parallel to the floor, and your stomach in. •Don't bounce or jerk. •Don't allow the weight to touch the floor. •Always put one hand on the bench to support your upper body and reduce the stress on your lower back. •Exhale through the upward movement and inhale during the downward movement.

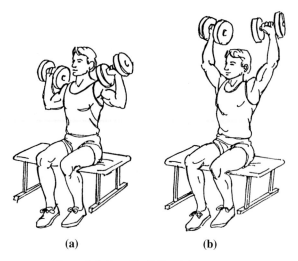

(a)   **(b)**

Figure 9-9. Dumbbell Shoulder Press

Muscles Used:	Deltoids, triceps
Starting Position:	Sit at end of bench with feet firmly on floor. Raise dumbbells to shoulder height. Keep palms facing forward, elbows out, and thumbs in. Keep back flat and hold stomach in.
Description:	Press dumbbells to arm's length overhead. Keep elbows pointed out to the sides until elbows are extended. Lower weights to shoulder height and then repeat.
Points to Emphasize:	•Maintain body position, do not lean from side to side or arch your back. •Hold your stomach in tight. •Do not forcefully lock out your elbows. •Exhale has you push the dumbbells up and inhale as you lower them. •This exercise can also be performed with a barbell.

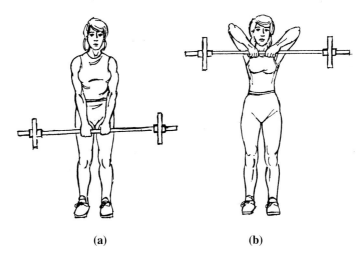

(a)   (b)

Figure 9-10. Barbell Upright Row

Muscles Used:	Deltoids, trapezius, biceps
Starting Position:	Grasp barbell in an overhand grip with hands placed 6-12 inches apart. Rest bar at arm's length on front of thighs. Assume a shoulder-width stance with knees slightly bent. Keep torso erect. Point elbows outward.
Description:	Pull bar upward along abdomen and chest towards chin. Keep bar very close to the torso. Keep torso erect. At top position, elbows are higher than wrists and above shoulders. Pause momentarily at top before lowering to starting position. Repeat upward pull.
Points to Emphasize:	•Do not jerk or swing the bar up.

•Do not bend forward at the waist or arch your back backward.
•Concentrate on your shoulders doing the work as you lower the weight.
•Exhale as you pull the weight up and inhale as it is lowered.
•This exercise can also be done with a wide grip or with dumbbells.

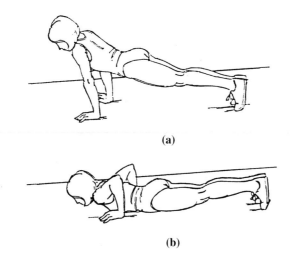

(a)

(b)

Figure 9-11. Push-up

Muscles Used:	Pectorals, deltoids, triceps
Starting Position:	From an all-fours position, extend and lock your knees to assume a front-leaning rest position. Place your palms wider than shoulder width. Keep your back straight and hold your stomach in.
Description:	With your body supported on your fully extended arms and toes, slowly lower your body to the floor by bending your elbows. The lowering movement should take two to three seconds. Once your body touches the floor, push yourself back into the starting position. Repeat the exercise.
Points to Emphasize:	•If the full position push-up is too difficult to begin with, a modification can be made: support your body on your extended arms and knees, with your feet held above the floor. Keep your shoulders, hips, and knees in a straight line, as to not allow your back to sway downward.
	•Maintain a flat back throughout the movement and keep your body rigid.
	•Exhale as you push up and inhale on the downward movement.

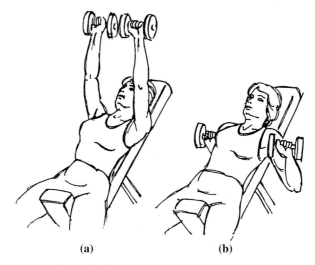

(a)   (b)

Figure 9-12. Dumbbell Incline Bench Press

Muscles Used:	Pectorals, deltoids, triceps
Starting Position:	Position head, shoulders, and buttocks flat on incline bench. Position feet flat on floor. Grasp dumbbells with a closed grip, palms facing forward. Press both dumbbells to extended arm position above your head. Point elbows out.
Description:	Lower dumbbells straight down to front of shoulders or outer chest. Keep forearms parallel. Maintain body position on bench, feet on floor. Push dumbbells to full elbow extension. Keep forearms parallel. Repeat using same path.
Points to Emphasize:	•Keep your head, shoulders, back, and hips flat on the bench. •Exhale when pushing the dumbbells up and inhale when lowering. •This exercise can also be performed on a flat or decline bench for variety. A barbell, rather than dumbbells can also be substituted.

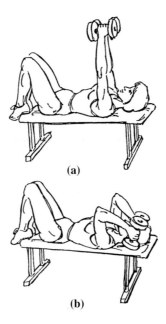

(a)

(b)

Figure 9-13. Lying Dumbbell Triceps Extension

Muscles Used:	Triceps
Starting Position:	Lie on your back on a bench. Grasp dumbbells at arm's length above shoulders. Position feet flat on floor or feet may be placed on the end of the bench to help support your lower back. Stomach should be held in tight.
Description:	Slowly lower dumbbells in a semicircular motion, bending arms at elbows until forearms touch biceps. Keeping upper arms perpendicular to floor. Dumbbells should come close to ears. Push dumbbells up until elbows are fully extended to return to starting position.
Points to Emphasize:	•Push the weight up by extending at the elbows only, do not use your shoulders to press the weight up.
	•Maintain body position on the bench with your back flat and your stomach held in.
	•Exhale as you press the dumbbells up and inhale as you lower the weight.
	•This exercise can also be done on the floor, or while seated upright on a bench.

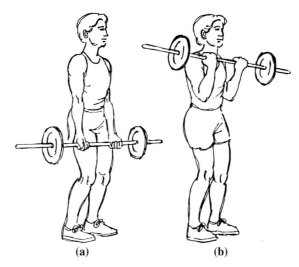

(a) (b)

Figure 9-14. Barbell Biceps Curl

Muscles Used:	Biceps
Starting Position:	Grasp the bar using a closed, underhand grip that is slightly wider than shoulder width. Little finger should be touching the outer thigh. Stand erect with feet shoulder-width apart, knees slightly bent. Place one foot four to eight inches in front of the other. Rest the bar on the upper thigh with your elbows fully extended. Upper arms should be held against the ribs perpendicular to floor.
Description:	Curl bar up in semicircular arc by flexing arms at the elbows until forearms touch biceps. Keep upper arms and elbows stationary and close to sides. Lower to starting position using same path. Repeat movement.
Points to Emphasize:	•Maintain a flat back and hold your stomach in throughout exercise.
	•Do not swing back and forth to help lift bar.
	•Exhale as you lift the weight and inhale as it is lowered.
	•This exercise can also be done with dumbbells or in the seated position.

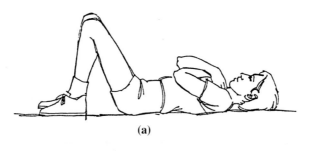

(a)

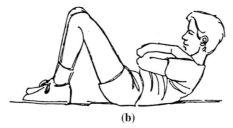

(b)

Figure 9-15. Bent-Knee Abdominal Crunch

Muscles Used:	Abdominals
Starting Position:	Lie face up on the mat or floor. Bring heels 12-16 inches to buttocks. Fold arms across chest or abdomen. Tuck chin to chest.
Description:	Curl upper body toward thighs until upper back is off mat. Keep feet flat on floor. Keep lower back flat on floor. Pause momentarily in the up position. To return, slowly lower your shoulders by controlling your abdominal muscles. Lower upper back to floor and with chin still tucked into chest, repeat another curl.
Points to Emphasize:	•Do not bounce or jerk your body.
	•Only raise your upper back off the floor.
	•Keep feet and lower back flat on the floor.
	•Press your lower back into the floor by tilting your hips forward and holding your stomach in.
	•Exhale as you curl up and inhale as you return down.

10. Stretch your muscles and increase your flexibility.

A lack of flexibility can lead to injuries and unnecessary muscle soreness. General stretching of the large muscle groups and those specifically used in an activity should be completed after the warm-up. Never try to stretch a cold muscle. Stretching a cold muscle is ineffective for increasing the elasticity of the muscle and, in itself, may lead to a soft tissue injury.

You will soon find that after your exercise session, when your muscles are thoroughly warmed-up, muscles are more supple and flexible. It is at this point in your workout that you are best able to increase the elasticity of the soft tissue.

FOR FLEXIBILITY

Mode: Slow, static stretches for the major muscle groups of the body.
Frequency: Daily preferred; at minimum on days that you exercise.
Duration: Hold each stretch 10-30 seconds.
Intensity: Stretch to a point of tension and feel a slight pull. Do not stretch to the point of pain.

FORMAT

Warm-up: Never stretch cold muscles. Warm-up with 5-10 minutes of an easy aerobic activity prior to performing flexibility exercises (if you are not already completing an aerobic exercise session).
Training: Stretching exercises should involve the head/neck, shoulders, back, thighs, and calves. Normal breathing should be maintained during stretching exercises. It is recommended that 3-5 sets of each exercise be performed.

Remember:
- Always stretch after your warm-up and cool-down sessions.
- The first one or two stretches should be very easy. You should feel mild tension through the muscle being stretched. The tension should decrease as you hold the position. The next two stretching repetitions should put slightly more tension on the muscle. Attempt to move further into the stretch, hold for 20-30 seconds.
- Hold stretches for a minimum of 10 seconds — preferably 20-30 seconds.
- Stretch to the point of mild tension, and relax as you hold the stretch.
- Never stretch to the point of pain.
- Never bounce or use jerky movements — make each movement smooth and controlled.

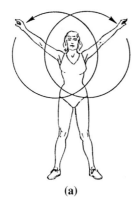 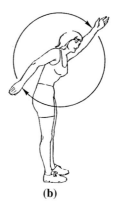

(a)   (b)

Figure 9-16. Arm Circles

- Stand with your feet apart, slightly wider than shoulder-width, knees slightly bent and arms at your side.
- On each of the following arm stretches, swing your arms slowly with large, sweeping circles. Swing your arms from the shoulders and keep your elbows straight.

(a) **Inward circles**:	Swing your arms inward, crossing in front of your body, moving upward, and over your head; repeat 10-15 times.
Outward circles:	Swing your arms outward, crossing in front of your body, moving upward, and over your head; repeat 10-15 times.
(b) **Forward circles**:	Swing your arms alternately forward, with large sweeping circles, as if swimming. Count one complete circle with the left and right arm as one repetition; repeat 10-15 times.
Backward circles:	Swing your arms alternately backward, with large sweeping circles. Count one complete circle with the left and right arm as one repetition; repeat 10-15 times.

108

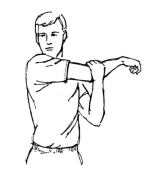

Figure 9-17. Shoulder Stretch

- Stand or sit with right arm across chest.
- Grasp the upper arm just above the elbow with the left hand.
- Gently pull the right arm further across the chest with the left hand.
- Do not rotate trunk in direction of stretch.
- Hold for 10-30 seconds.
- Repeat with left arm, relax, repeat two to three times with each arm.

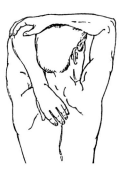

Figure 9-18. Triceps Stretch

- Standing or sitting, raise left arm over head.
- Bend at elbow and place left hand on back between shoulder blades.
- Grasp left elbow with right hand.
- Gently pull left elbow behind head and downward.
- Hold for 10-30 seconds.
- Repeat with right arm, relax, repeat two to three times with each arm.

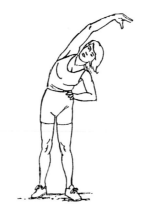

Figure 9-19. Side Stretch

•Stand with feet apart, slightly wider than shoulder-width, knees slightly bent, and toes
  pointing straight ahead.
•Place left hand on left hip for support.
•Lift right arm up in line with right ear and reach upward as high as possible.
•Continue the stretch by arching the torso further to the left. Be sure to stretch from the
  side and not twist at the waist.
•Hold for 10-30 seconds.
•Return arms to side and repeat with left arm overhead; relax, repeat two to three times
  each arm.

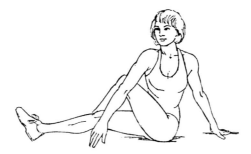

Figure 9-20. Hip Twist and Gluteal Stretch

•Sitting with legs straight and upper body nearly vertical, place left foot on right side of
  right knee.
•Place back of right elbow on left side of left knee, which is now bent.
•Stabilize your upper body with your left hand placed 12-18 inches behind your left hip.
•Gently push left knee to the right with the right elbow while turning shoulders and head
  to the left as far as possible.
•Hold for 10-20 seconds.
•Repeat with right leg, relax, repeat two to three times for each side.

110

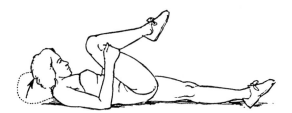

Figure 9-21. Lower Back and Gluteal Stretch

- Lie on back while pressing lower back to floor with both legs extended.
- Bend right knee, grasp behind your knee and pull towards chest, while keeping head on floor.
- Hold for a count of five, then curl shoulders and lift upper head and shoulders toward knee.
- Hold for five seconds.
- Lower shoulders and then lower right leg back to floor and repeat with left leg, relax, repeat two to three times for each leg.

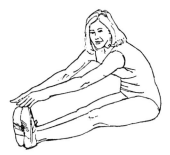

Figure 9-22. Hamstring Stretch

- Sit with both legs extended in front, with the back of your knees touching the floor, toes pointed up.
- Slowly lean forward from your waist, sliding the palms of your hands along the side of your legs.
- Keep your back straight and lean forward from the hips.
- Keep you eyes focused comfortably forward with your head naturally bent down; do not strain your neck to look up.
- Try to grasp toes with each hand, slightly pull toes towards the upper body, and pull chest towards legs. (If you are very stiff, try to grasp your ankles.)
- Release toes and relax feet.
- Grasp ankles and continue to pull chest toward legs.
- Hold for 10-30 seconds.
- Sit up and relax, repeat two to three times for each leg.

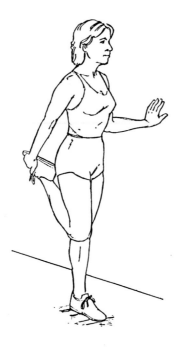

Figure 9-23. Quadriceps Stretch

- Stand on left leg, holding onto wall or fixed object with left hand.
- Bend right knee and grasp right ankle with right hand, knee pointing down.
- Slowly pull right heel towards buttocks. Do not pull on ankle so hard that pain or discomfort is felt in knee.
- Keep back flat and stand tall.
- Move knee backward and slightly upward. The stretch occurs not so much from the excessive flexing of the knee, but from moving the knee behind the upper torso and slightly up.
- Hold for 10-30 seconds.
- Repeat with the left leg, relax; repeat two to three times for each leg.

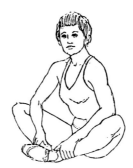

Figure 9-24. Groin Stretch

- Sitting with the upper body nearly vertical and legs straight, bend both knees as the soles of the feet come together.
- Grasp ankles and pull feet towards body.
- Place hands on feet and elbows on thighs.
- While keeping back flat, pull torso slightly forward as elbows push thighs down.
- Hold for 10-15 seconds, relax; repeat two to three times.

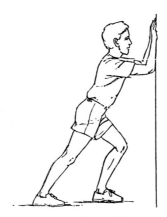

Figure 9-25. Calf Stretch

- Stand facing a wall or other solid support. Place outstretched hands or forearms on wall.
- Place right leg behind the left leg, keeping right leg straight.
- Slowly move your hips and upper torso forward, keeping your back flat, and the heel of rear foot on ground.
- Hold stretch for 10-20 seconds.
- Slowly begin to lower your body a few inches by bending the right knee and keeping the heel of the rear foot on ground.
- Hold for 10-20 seconds
- Repeat with the left leg behind the right, relax; repeat two to three times for each leg.

YOUR EXERCISE PROGRAM

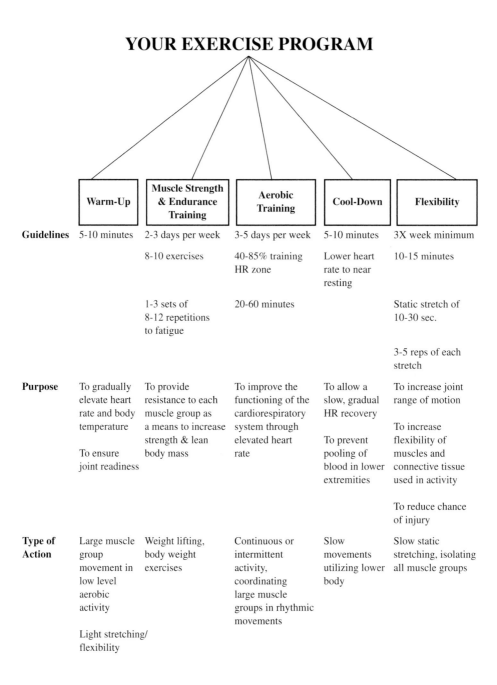

	Warm-Up	Muscle Strength & Endurance Training	Aerobic Training	Cool-Down	Flexibility
Guidelines	5-10 minutes	2-3 days per week	3-5 days per week	5-10 minutes	3X week minimum
		8-10 exercises	40-85% training HR zone	Lower heart rate to near resting	10-15 minutes
		1-3 sets of 8-12 repetitions to fatigue	20-60 minutes		Static stretch of 10-30 sec.
					3-5 reps of each stretch
Purpose	To gradually elevate heart rate and body temperature	To provide resistance to each muscle group as a means to increase strength & lean body mass	To improve the functioning of the cardiorespiratory system through elevated heart rate	To allow a slow, gradual HR recovery	To increase joint range of motion
	To ensure joint readiness			To prevent pooling of blood in lower extremities	To increase flexibility of muscles and connective tissue used in activity
					To reduce chance of injury
Type of Action	Large muscle group movement in low level aerobic activity	Weight lifting, body weight exercises	Continuous or intermittent activity, coordinating large muscle groups in rhythmic movements	Slow movements utilizing lower body	Slow static stretching, isolating all muscle groups
	Light stretching/ flexibility				

Conclusion

In this chapter we have given you a complete and detailed exercise program. If it seems overwhelming, don't be discouraged. Start slowly and progress gradually — listen to your body. Develop a routine that fits your lifestyle and take one day at a time. Make exercise fun and simple and it can easily become a part of your life. Instead of taking an elevator up one floor, walk up the stairs. After three to four weeks, you may be able to walk up two flights of stairs with ease. Park your car a block or two from the store and enjoy the walk outdoors. Walk or ride a bike to work. Combine a walk with a stretch break at lunch time. The key is to increase your activity level on a daily basis. It will surprise you how many opportunities you have in your everyday activities to increase your amount of daily activity. Keep in mind the counsel of the NIH Panel and encourage family and friends, both adults and children, to accumulate at least 30 minutes of moderate-intensity physical activity every day of the week. The increase in activity by members of all generations will improve the health and well-being of all Americans (NIH Panel, 1996).

Use this chapter to guide you in your exercise program. More than anything else, start a program today, no matter how simple and have fun.

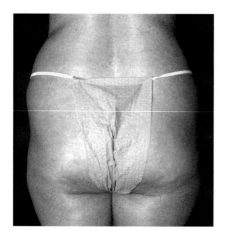 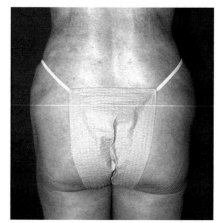

Used with permission, C. William Hanke, M.D.

References

The American Cancer Society 1996 Advisory Committee: Guidelines on Diet, Nutrition, and Cancer Prevention: Reducing the risk of cancer with healthy food choices and physical activity. *CA Cancer J Clin 1996;* 46:325-341.

Bernstein G, Hanke CW: Safety of liposuction. A review of 9,478 cases performed by dermatologists. *J Dermatol Surg Oncol* 1988; 14:1112-1114.

Coleman WP III: The history of liposuction surgery, In Lillis PG (ed): *Dermatology Clinics,* vol 8. Philadelphia, WB Saunders, 1990; pp 381-383.

Coleman WP III: Liposuction. In *Cosmetic Surgery of the Skin* (Coleman WP, Hanke CW, Alt TH, Asken S - eds), Philadelphia, BC Decker, 1991; pp 213-238.

Coleman WP III: Liposuction. *In Cutaneous Surgery* (Wheeland R - ed), Philadelphia, WB Saunders, 1994; pp 549-567.

Coleman WP III: Fat transplantation. *Dermatol Clin* 17:4 pp 891-898, 1999.

Coleman WP III: Powered liposuction. *Dermatol Surg* 2000; 26:315-318

Coleman WP III, Glogau R, Klein JA, Moy RL, Narins RS, Chuang TY, Farmer ER, Lewis CW, Lowery BJ: Guidelines of Care for Liposuction. *J Am Acad Dermatol.* 2001; 45:438-47.

Coleman WP III, Katz BE, Bruck M, Narins R, Lawrence N, Flynn T, Coleman, WP IV, Coleman, K: The efficacy of powered liposuction *Dermatol Surg.* 2001; 27:235-8.

Cook WR: "Three-dimensional tumescent liposculpture of the abdomen, waist, and flanks." In: Coleman WP and Lillis PJ (eds) : *Dermatologic Clinics on Liposuction. Dermatol Clin.* 17:805-813 1999.

Field L: The dermatologist and liposuction history. *J Dermatol Surg Oncol* 1987; 13:1040-1041.

Fischer G: Liposculpture: The "correct" history of liposuction. *J Dermatol Surg Oncol* 1990; 16:1087-1089.

Flynn TC, Coleman WP, Field LM, Klein JA, Hanke CW: History of liposuction *Dermatol Surg* 2000; 26:515-520.

Hanke CW, Bernstein G, Bullock S: Safety of tumescent liposuction in 15,336 patients. *J Dermatol Surg Oncol* 1995; 21:459-462.

Hanke CW, Bullock S, Bernstein G: Current status of tumescent liposuction in the United States. *Dermatol Surg.* 1996; 22:595-598.

Hanke CW, Coleman WP, Lillis PJ et al: Infusion rates and levels of premedication in tumescent liposuction *Dermatol Surg 1997;* 23: 1131-1134.

Hanke, CW, Sommer B, Sattler G: Tumescent Local Anesthesia. Berlin. Springer. 2002.

Houseman TS, Lawrence N, Mellen BG et al: The safety of liposuction: results of a national survey. *Dermatol Surg* 2002; 28:971-978.

Katz BR, Bruck MC, Coleman WP III: The benefits of powered liposuction vs traditional liposuction: a paired comparison analysis. *Dermatol Surg* 2001; 27:863-7

Klein JA: The tumescent technique for liposuction surgery. *Am J Cosmet Surg* 1987; 4:263-267.

Klein JA: Tumescent technique for regional anesthesia permits lidocaine doses of 35 mg/kg for liposuction: peak plasma levels are diminished and delayed 12 hours. J *Dermatol Surg* Oncol 1990; 16:248- 263.

Klein JA: Tumescent technique for local anesthesia improves safety in large-volume liposuction. *Plast Reconstr Surg* 1993; 92:1085-1098.

Klein JA: Tumescent Technique-Tumescent Anesthesia & Microcannular Liposuction. St. Louis. Mosby, 2000.

Lawrence N, Coleman WP III: Liposuction (periodic synopsis) *J Am Acad Dermatol* 2002; 47:105-8.

Lillis PJ: Liposuction surgery under local anesthesia: limited blood loss and minimal lidocaine absorption. *J Dermatol Surg Oncol* 1988; 14:1145-1148.

Narins RS: Liposuction surgery for a buffalo hump, caused by Cushing's disease. *JAAD* 1989; 21:307.

Narins RS: *Cosmetic Surgery: An Interdisciplinary Approach,* New York. Marcel Dekker Inc, 2000.

Narins RS: Safe Liposuction and Fat Transfer, Marcel Dekker, New York, 2003.

Physical Activity and Cardiovascular Health, NIH Consensus Development Panel. *JAMA* 1996; 276:241-246.

Physical Activity and Health, A Report of the Surgeon General, US Department of Health and Human Services, 1996.

References

Skouge JW: The biochemistry and development of adipose tissue and pathophysiology of obesity as it relates to liposuction surgery, *Dermatology Clinics*, (Lillis PJ - ed), vol 8, no 3. Philadelphia, WB Saunders pp. 385-393, 1990.

US Department of Agriculture (USDA) and US Department of Health and Human Services. Nutrition and your Health: Dietary guidelines for Americans, 4th ed; 1995.